Super Easy

METABOLIC CONFUSION

Diet Cookbook

for

Endomorph Women Over 50

The Proven 6-Week Plan to Balance Hormones and Burn Stubborn Fat with Quick, Delicious, and Affordable 5-Ingredient Recipes

Cynthia Digges

Copyright © 2025 Super Easy Metabolic Confusion Diet Cookbook for Endomorph Women Over 50

By Cynthia Digges

All rights reserved. This book is for informational purposes only. Unauthorized copying or sharing, in whole or part, is prohibited. All trademarks and brand names are owned by their respective holders. The publisher is not liable for any damages from the use or misuse of this information. This book is provided 'as is' without any warranties, either express or implied.

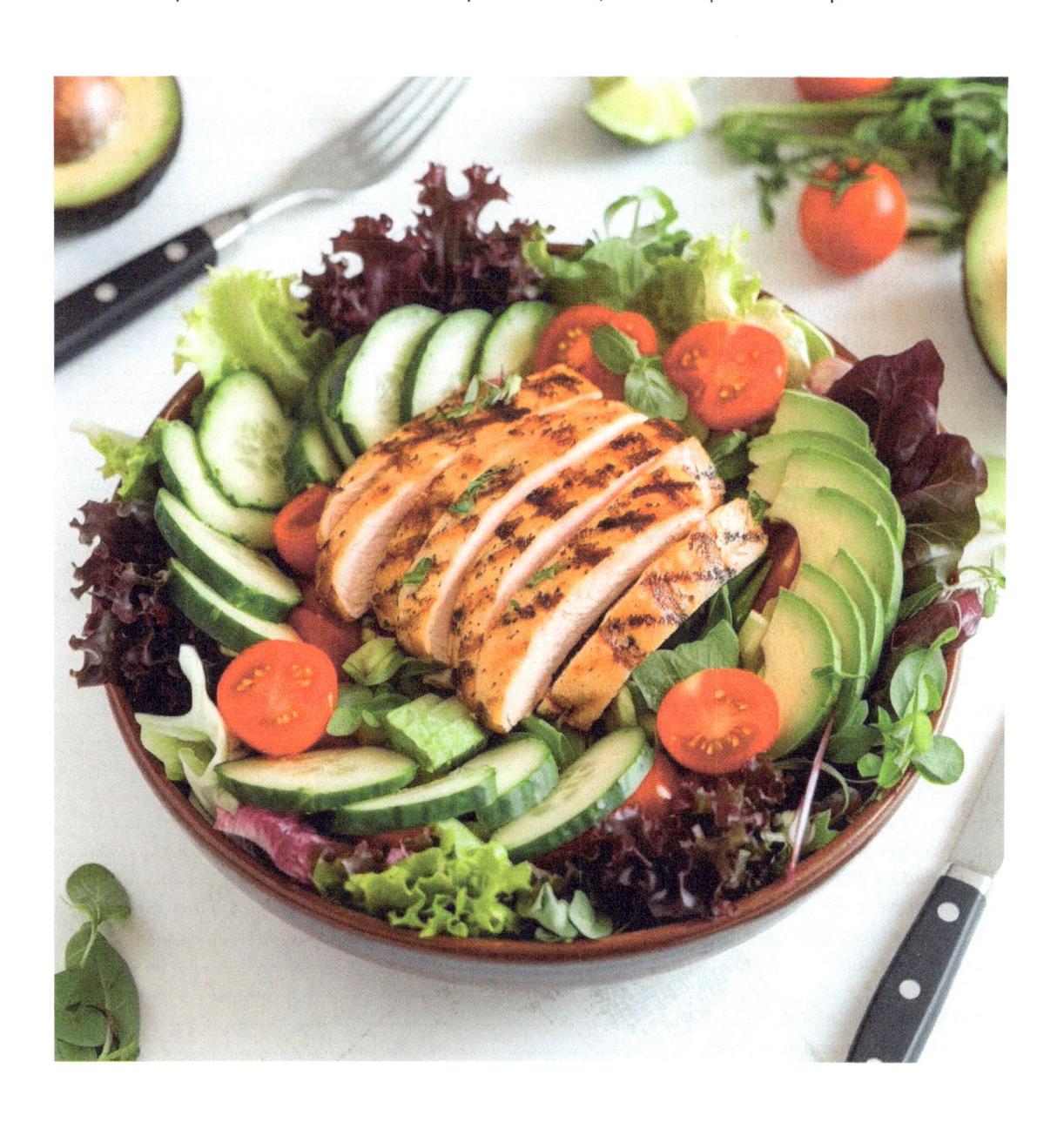

TABLE OF CONTENTS

FOREWORD FROM THE AUTHOR 1

INTRODUCTION: A NEW BEGINNING FOR WOMEN OVER 50 2
   How This Book Will Help You 2

CHAPTER 1: UNDERSTANDING YOUR ENDOMORPH BODY TYPE 4
   What It Means to Be an Endomorph Woman Over 50 4
   Common Weight Loss Struggles for Endomorphs 5

CHAPTER 2: THE SCIENCE OF METABOLIC CONFUSION 7
   What Is the Metabolic Confusion Diet? 7
   How Calorie Cycling Boosts Fat Loss and Prevents Plateaus 8

CHAPTER 3: THE 5-INGREDIENT RECIPES 10

CHAPTER 4: HIGH-CALORIE DAY RECIPES 11
   High-Calorie Breakfasts 11
      1. Avocado and Bacon Breakfast Wrap 11
      2. Peanut Butter Banana Oatmeal 11
      3. Ricotta and Berry Stuffed French Toast 12
      4. Spinach and Cheese Omelette 12
      5. Smoked Salmon and Cream Cheese Bagel 13
      6. Almond Butter and Honey Pancakes 13
      7. Sausage and Egg Breakfast Bowl 14
      8. Cheddar and Ham Breakfast Quesadilla 14
      9. Greek Yogurt and Granola Parfait 15
      10. Mushroom and Swiss Cheese Frittata 15
      11. Chia Seed Pudding with Mixed Nuts 16
      12. Turkey and Avocado Breakfast Sandwich 16
   High-Calorie Lunch Recipes 17
      13. Grilled Chicken and Avocado Salad 17
      14. Quinoa and Black Bean Burrito Bowl 17
      15. Shrimp and Spinach Stir-Fry 18
      16. Beef and Broccoli Power Bowl 18
      17. Turkey and Sweet Potato Skillet 19
      18. Chicken and Quinoa Stuffed Peppers 19
      19. Lentil and Kale Soup 20
      20. Tuna and White Bean Salad 20
      21. Steak and Arugula Wrap 21
      22. Sesame Ginger Salmon Bowl 21
      23. Chicken and Zucchini Noodles 22
      24. Pork and Apple Slaw 22
      25. Balsamic Mushroom and Spinach Pasta 23
      26. Spicy Chickpea and Tomato Stew 23
   High-Calorie Dinners 24
      27. Grilled Steak with Chimichurri Sauce 24
      28. Creamy Shrimp Alfredo with Spinach 24
      29. Honey Garlic Pork Chops 25
      30. Chicken Alfredo with Broccoli 25
      31. Stuffed Bell Peppers with Ground Beef 26
      32. Maple Glazed Salmon with Quinoa 26
      33. Beef Stroganoff with Mushrooms 27
      34. BBQ Chicken Thighs with Sweet Potatoes 27

35. Lemon Herb Roasted Chicken with Asparagus 28
36. Pork Tenderloin with Apples and Onions 28
37. Shrimp Scampi with Zoodles 29
38. Teriyaki Beef Stir-Fry 29

High-Calorie Snacks 30
39. Trail Mix Energy Bars 30
40. Apple and Almond Butter Bites 30
41. Coconut Cashew Clusters 31
42. Dark Chocolate Walnut Bites 31
43. Greek Yogurt with Honey and Pecans 32
44. Peanut Butter and Jelly Protein Balls 32
45. Cheese and Sun-Dried Tomato Crackers 33
46. Avocado Hummus with Pita Chips 33
47. Banana and Nutella Roll-Ups 34
48. Roasted Chickpeas with Parmesan 34
49. Almond and Cranberry Rice Cakes 35
50. Sweet Potato and Black Bean Nachos 35

CHAPTER 5: LOW-CALORIE DAY RECIPES 36

Low-Calorie Breakfasts 36
51. Blueberry Almond Overnight Oats 36
52. Egg White and Spinach Scramble 36
53. Cottage Cheese with Pineapple 37
54. Tomato and Feta Cheese Muffins 37
55. Cucumber and Cream Cheese Roll-Ups 38
56. Apple Cinnamon Smoothie 38
57. Avocado and Tomato Toast 39
58. Berry and Chia Seed Smoothie 39
59. Egg and Avocado Breakfast Wrap 40
60. Zucchini and Tomato Frittata 40
61. Raspberry and Yogurt Parfait 41
62. Peach and Walnut Smoothie 41

Low-Calorie Lunches 42
63. Grilled Vegetable and Quinoa Salad 42
64. Lemon Herb Tofu Wrap 42
65. Cucumber and Turkey Roll-Ups 43
66. Spinach and Feta Lettuce Wraps 43
67. Tuna and Cucumber Salad 44
68. Egg and Tomato Salad 44
69. Zucchini and Hummus Wrap 45
70. Chicken and Avocado Lettuce Wrap 45
71. Cottage Cheese and Cucumber Bowl 46
72. Broccoli and Cheese Stuffed Peppers 46
73. Tomato and Basil Salad 47
74. Carrot and Hummus Roll-Ups 47
75. Eggplant and Tomato Stack 48
76. Cauliflower Rice Stir-Fry 48

Low-Calorie Dinners 49
77. Grilled Lemon Herb Chicken Breast 49
78. Baked Cod with Garlic and Lemon 49
79. Spaghetti Squash with Marinara Sauce 50
80. Garlic Lime Shrimp Skewers 50
81. Turkey and Spinach Stuffed Bell Peppers 51
82. Zucchini Noodles with Pesto 51
83. Grilled Portobello Mushroom Caps 52

84. Lemon Dill Baked Salmon 52
85. Chicken and Asparagus Stir-Fry 53
86. Cauliflower and Chickpea Curry 53
87. Balsamic Glazed Tofu with Vegetables 54
88. Cilantro Lime Grilled Chicken 54

Low-Calorie Snacks 55
89. Cucumber and Avocado Bites 55
90. Spicy Tuna Lettuce Cups 55
91. Roasted Red Pepper Hummus Dip 56
92. Apple and Peanut Butter Slices 56
93. Celery Sticks with Cream Cheese 57
94. Cherry Tomato and Basil Skewers 57
95. Almond Butter Stuffed Dates 58
96. Mini Caprese Salad Cups 58
97. Kale Chips with Sea Salt 59
98. Bell Pepper and Hummus Boats 59
99. Greek Yogurt with Berries 60
100. Edamame with Sea Salt 60

CHAPTER 6: THE 6-WEEK METABOLIC CONFUSION PLAN 61
How to Structure a Week with Calorie Cycling 61
Customizing the Plan for Your Lifestyle 63
The 6-Week Meal Plan 65

CHAPTER 7: TAILORING YOUR CALORIE PLAN FOR MAXIMUM RESULTS 70

CHAPTER 8: OVERCOMING CHALLENGES AND THRIVING BEYOND THE 6-WEEK PLAN 72

CONCLUSION 73

Foreword from the author

I'll be honest with you—writing this book felt deeply personal. As an endomorph woman over 50, I've lived through the struggles this book aims to address. I've felt the frustration of diets that seem to work for everyone else but me. I've experienced the discouragement of stepping on the scale and seeing no change despite my best efforts. I've battled with the stubborn fat that clings to the hips, thighs, and belly, no matter how disciplined I tried to be. And yes, I've worried about the effects of hormonal imbalances, low energy, and the toll that weight gain can take on my overall health and mobility.

This book isn't just another cookbook. It's my response to those challenges and unmet needs that I know so many women like me experience. I've been exactly where you are, feeling overwhelmed by conflicting advice—"cut carbs," "go keto," "try fasting"—all of it confusing and, in many cases, unsustainable. After years of searching for the right approach, I discovered the concept of metabolic confusion, and it changed everything for me.

Unlike the rigid, restrictive diets that left me drained, metabolic confusion brought something new—flexibility and freedom. By alternating between low and high-calorie days, I learned how to trick my body into burning fat efficiently while avoiding the dreaded weight-loss plateaus. I didn't feel deprived. I wasn't constantly hungry. And for the first time in years, I had energy. I could focus on my family, enjoy my favorite activities, and stop obsessing over what I could and couldn't eat.

But I didn't stop there. I knew that to make this lifestyle truly sustainable, it had to be simple, practical, and affordable. That's why this book focuses on 5-ingredient recipes that anyone can prepare—whether you're an experienced cook or someone who prefers quick meals without the fuss. I wanted to create something that wouldn't require hours in the kitchen or expensive, hard-to-find ingredients. Instead, you'll find everyday meals that nourish your body and fit into your life seamlessly.

This journey isn't just about losing weight. It's about feeling good in your skin, restoring your energy, balancing your hormones, and creating a healthier future. It's about finally having a plan that works with your body's natural tendencies instead of fighting against them.

So, if you've ever felt defeated by diets that didn't deliver or if you've wondered if it's even possible to lose weight after 50, I'm here to tell you—it is. You are not alone in this, and you're not doomed to struggle forever. With the right plan, you can experience real results without sacrificing your joy or freedom.

This book is my gift to women like you—women who have spent too long searching for answers and deserve a solution that's sustainable, science-backed, and designed specifically for them. Let's navigate this journey together.

Cynthia Digges

Introduction: A New Beginning for Women Over 50

Welcome to a fresh start, designed just for you. As an endomorph woman over 50, you've likely faced challenges that most diets simply don't address—hormonal changes, slower metabolism, and stubborn fat that doesn't seem to budge. But here's the truth: your body isn't working against you. With the right approach, it can become your greatest ally. The Metabolic Confusion Diet isn't about restriction; it's about flexibility, balance, and simplicity. This book combines proven science with easy, 5-ingredient recipes to empower you with the tools you need to feel healthier, more energized, and in control of your weight—starting today.

How This Book Will Help You

As an endomorph woman over 50, your journey to better health and weight loss might feel like an uphill battle. This isn't because you lack willpower or discipline; it's because most diets fail to address the unique needs of your body type and the natural changes that come with age. This book is designed to meet you exactly where you are, with a plan tailored to your specific needs. Here's how this cookbook will transform your approach to health, step by step:

1. Burn Fat Without Feeling Deprived

Weight loss doesn't have to mean giving up the foods you love or enduring constant hunger. The Metabolic Confusion Diet uses a strategic calorie-cycling approach that keeps your metabolism active and fat-burning, while allowing for satisfying high-calorie days. With this book, you'll learn how to alternate low-calorie and high-calorie days in a way that works with your body's natural rhythms, helping you shed stubborn fat without feeling like you're on a diet.

2. Balance Hormones Naturally

Hormonal changes after 50—like fluctuations in estrogen, insulin sensitivity, and cortisol—can make weight loss more challenging and lead to low energy, mood swings, and increased fat storage. This book goes beyond recipes; it provides you with actionable nutrition strategies designed to naturally balance your hormones. By choosing the right foods on both high- and low-calorie days, you'll support hormone regulation, reduce inflammation, and set the stage for sustainable weight loss.

3. Boost Your Energy with Nutrient-Packed Meals

Feeling tired and sluggish isn't just a side effect of aging—it's often a result of poor nutrition. The recipes in this cookbook are carefully crafted with nutrient-dense ingredients that nourish your body and stabilize blood sugar levels. By focusing on simple, 5-ingredient meals, you'll save time in the kitchen while fueling your body for an energetic and vibrant lifestyle.

4. Save Time and Money with Simple Recipes

You don't need a pantry full of exotic ingredients or hours in the kitchen to see results. Each recipe in this book is designed to be quick, affordable, and made with only 5 ingredients. This makes it easy to stay consistent, even on your busiest days, while also reducing the stress of meal planning. With this approach, healthy eating becomes a joy—not a chore.

5. Break Through Plateaus with Flexibility

Most diets fail because they're too rigid, leading to burnout and frustration. The Metabolic Confusion Diet allows for flexibility, making it easier to stick with long-term. This book teaches you how to adjust your plan based on your lifestyle and preferences, so you can keep progressing without feeling restricted or overwhelmed.

6. Build Habits for Lifelong Health

This isn't just another quick-fix diet—it's a guide to creating a lifestyle that supports your health and happiness well beyond six weeks. You'll learn tips for mindful eating, portion control without calorie counting, and ways to make these strategies part of your daily life. By the end of this book, you'll have the tools and confidence to maintain your results and thrive in your healthiest years yet.

With this cookbook as your guide, you'll discover that losing weight, balancing hormones, and boosting energy isn't about perfection—it's about finding what works for you. Let this be the starting point for a healthier, happier you, free from the frustration of diets that don't deliver. You've got this!

Chapter 1: Understanding Your Endomorph Body Type

Your body is unique, and understanding how it works is the first step toward lasting weight loss and better health. As an endomorph, your body is naturally predisposed to storing fat, especially in areas like the hips, thighs, and abdomen. This can make traditional diets feel ineffective and frustrating. But here's the good news: your body type isn't a limitation—it's your guide. By learning how to work *with* your body instead of against it, you'll unlock the tools to burn fat more efficiently, balance your hormones, and feel your best. Let's explore what makes your body type so special!

What It Means to Be an Endomorph Woman Over 50

Being an endomorph woman over 50 comes with unique challenges—but also unique strengths. Understanding how your body type functions and responds to nutrition, exercise, and hormonal changes is key to unlocking sustainable weight loss and a healthier, more vibrant life.

1. The Traits of an Endomorph Body Type

Endomorphs tend to have a naturally curvier, softer body shape, with a predisposition to store fat more easily than other body types. Common characteristics include:

- A wider waist and hips compared to shoulders.
- A slower metabolic rate, making weight loss more difficult.
- Sensitivity to carbohydrates, which can quickly be stored as fat if not balanced with protein and fats.
  These traits are not flaws—they're simply part of how your body is built. With the right strategies, you can harness these tendencies to your advantage.

2. How Aging Impacts Endomorph Women

After the age of 50, natural hormonal changes, like a decline in estrogen and progesterone, can further slow metabolism and increase fat storage. Muscle mass tends to decrease, which can exacerbate the feeling of "stubborn" weight that doesn't seem to shift.

These changes may also bring:

- Increased insulin resistance, making it harder to process sugars and carbs.
- A tendency to retain water and feel bloated.
- Slower recovery after exercise or illness.

However, these shifts don't mean weight loss is impossible—it just requires an approach tailored to your body's needs.

3. Why Diets Often Fail for Endomorph Women

If you've tried diet after diet with little success, you're not alone. Traditional low-calorie or one-size-fits-all plans don't account for the way endomorph bodies store fat or respond to food. Common frustrations include:

- Feeling hungry and deprived on low-calorie diets that neglect the need for healthy fats and proteins.
- Difficulty losing weight despite strict dieting, due to an already slower metabolism.
- Rapid weight gain when returning to "normal" eating patterns.

The problem isn't your body—it's the diet. To see real results, you need a plan that works with your natural tendencies instead of fighting them.

4. Embracing Your Strengths as an Endomorph Woman

It's important to recognize the unique advantages of your body type:

- **Efficient fat storage:** This isn't just a challenge—it's also a survival trait! Your body is excellent at preserving energy, which means with the right balance, you'll see faster results when you begin burning fat.
- **Adaptability to change:** Endomorphs respond well to structured plans, especially those like the Metabolic Confusion Diet, which breaks weight-loss plateaus.
- **Strong, curvy physique:** When paired with the right nutrition and exercise, endomorphs can develop lean muscle and a balanced figure that radiates health and confidence.

5. What You'll Learn in This Book

This chapter is the foundation for everything to come. As you continue through the book, you'll learn how to tailor your meals, manage calorie cycling, and use your body's natural tendencies to your advantage. You'll discover the power of foods that stabilize blood sugar, balance hormones, and boost energy—all while embracing the beauty of your unique body type.

Being an endomorph woman over 50 isn't a limitation—it's an opportunity to approach weight loss and health in a way that's truly aligned with your body.

Common Weight Loss Struggles for Endomorphs

If you're an endomorph woman, especially over 50, the weight loss journey can feel uniquely frustrating. You're not alone in facing these challenges—they're a natural part of how your body processes food, stores energy, and reacts to hormonal changes. The good news? Understanding these struggles is the first step toward overcoming them.

1. Your Metabolism Works Differently

Endomorphs naturally have a slower metabolic rate, meaning your body burns fewer calories at rest compared to other body types. This isn't a flaw; it's simply how your body conserves energy. However, it can make traditional calorie-restriction diets less effective because:

- Severe calorie cutting can slow your metabolism even further.
- Extended low-calorie diets often lead to plateaus, where your body holds onto fat for survival.

Solution: The Metabolic Confusion Diet offers a way to "wake up" your metabolism with calorie cycling, helping your body burn fat without the drawbacks of traditional dieting.

2. Sensitivity to Carbohydrates

As an endomorph, your body is more likely to store carbs as fat rather than burning them for energy. This sensitivity can lead to:

- Weight gain, especially in the hips, thighs, and abdomen.
- Blood sugar spikes and crashes that cause cravings and fatigue.

This doesn't mean carbs are the enemy—it just means you need the right balance. By alternating low-calorie and high-calorie days, paired with strategic carb intake, you can stabilize blood sugar and prevent the dreaded carb-related weight gain.

3. Hormonal Changes After 50

Hormonal shifts during menopause, including declining levels of estrogen and progesterone, significantly impact weight loss for endomorph women. These changes can result in:

- Increased fat storage around the midsection.
- Difficulty building or maintaining muscle, which is key to burning fat.
- Slower recovery from exercise and reduced energy levels.

Solution: The Metabolic Confusion Diet prioritizes nutrient-dense foods that support hormonal balance, reduce inflammation, and help you regain control over your weight.

4. Emotional Eating and Cravings

Endomorphs are often more susceptible to emotional eating, especially when dealing with the stresses of everyday life or the challenges of aging. Common triggers include:

- Stress, leading to a reliance on comfort foods.
- Feelings of deprivation from overly restrictive diets.
- A cycle of guilt and frustration when cravings take over.

Solution: This book includes simple, 5-ingredient recipes that are satisfying and delicious, so you'll never feel deprived. Plus, the flexibility of the plan allows you to enjoy your favorite foods in moderation.

5. Weight Loss Plateaus

Many endomorph women experience the dreaded plateau—losing some weight initially, only for progress to stall. This happens because your body is incredibly adaptive and adjusts to prolonged calorie deficits by slowing your metabolism.

- Plateaus can be discouraging, often leading to giving up.
- Most diets don't offer solutions to "reset" your body and push past these roadblocks.

Solution: The Metabolic Confusion Diet is specifically designed to prevent plateaus by alternating calorie intake, keeping your metabolism guessing and active.

6. Lack of Time and Energy

Between busy schedules, family responsibilities, and the natural energy dips that come with age, finding the time and motivation to stick to a diet plan can feel impossible.

- Complicated meal prep and restrictive diets often feel overwhelming.
- Low energy can make cooking or exercise seem like a chore.

Solution: This cookbook focuses on quick, affordable, and easy-to-make recipes using just 5 ingredients. By simplifying meal prep, it removes one of the biggest barriers to staying consistent.

Why These Struggles Aren't Permanent

Every challenge you face as an endomorph woman has a solution. Your body isn't broken—it just requires a smarter, more tailored approach. This book is here to help you understand those challenges and equip you with the tools to overcome them. You'll discover strategies to manage carbs, balance hormones, and break through plateaus, all while enjoying delicious meals that make healthy eating a joy.

You're not just starting another diet—you're embarking on a path to understanding and working with your body for lasting health and confidence. Let's tackle these struggles together!

Chapter 2: The Science of Metabolic Confusion

Your metabolism is like a finely tuned machine, but as an endomorph woman over 50, you may feel like it's working against you. That's where metabolic confusion comes in—a flexible, science-backed approach designed to reset your metabolism and keep it working efficiently. By alternating between high-calorie and low-calorie days, this strategy prevents the metabolic slowdown that often sabotages weight loss. Think of it as giving your metabolism a wake-up call, helping your body burn fat without hitting frustrating plateaus. In this chapter, we'll dive into the science behind this powerful method and how it's perfectly suited to your needs.

What Is the Metabolic Confusion Diet?

The Metabolic Confusion Diet is a revolutionary approach to weight loss that's designed to work *with* your body, not against it. Unlike traditional diets that rely on strict calorie restriction, this method alternates between high-calorie and low-calorie days, keeping your metabolism engaged and adaptable. For women over 50, especially those with an endomorph body type, this is a game-changer.

How Does It Work?

At its core, the Metabolic Confusion Diet is all about calorie cycling—shifting your daily caloric intake to "confuse" your metabolism. Here's the idea: when your body gets used to the same low-calorie intake day after day, your metabolism slows down to conserve energy. This makes it harder to lose weight over time, leading to frustrating plateaus.

With metabolic confusion:

- **High-Calorie Days:** Fuel your body, replenish glycogen stores, and provide the energy needed for active days.
- **Low-Calorie Days:** Create a calorie deficit to burn fat without depriving your body.

By alternating between these two phases, your metabolism stays active and responsive, making fat loss more efficient and sustainable.

Why Is It Perfect for Women Over 50?

As women age, hormonal changes and a slower metabolism can make weight loss feel nearly impossible. The Metabolic Confusion Diet directly addresses these challenges:

- **Prevents Metabolic Slowdowns:** Keeps your resting metabolic rate (RMR) steady, so you burn more calories even at rest.
- **Balances Hormones Naturally:** Supports insulin regulation and reduces cortisol spikes, which are common after menopause.
- **Provides Flexibility:** Allows for variety and enjoyment in your meals, making it easier to stay consistent over time.

This approach isn't about perfection—it's about progress, designed to meet your body where it is today.

A Flexible Approach for Real Life

One of the standout benefits of the Metabolic Confusion Diet is its flexibility. You don't have to follow a rigid schedule or count every calorie. Instead, it's about creating a sustainable rhythm that fits your lifestyle. For example:

- On busy, active days, you enjoy higher-calorie meals that fuel your energy.
- On slower, less active days, you opt for lighter, low-calorie options that encourage fat burning.

This adaptability makes it especially practical for women juggling work, family, or simply enjoying a well-earned slower pace of life.

The Science Behind the Success

Metabolic confusion isn't just a trendy term—it's backed by real science. Studies show that calorie cycling can:

1. **Enhance Fat Loss:** By keeping your metabolism engaged, you avoid the "starvation mode" that stalls progress.
2. **Improve Diet Adherence:** The inclusion of high-calorie days makes it easier to stick with the plan without feeling deprived.
3. **Support Muscle Retention:** Unlike extreme calorie restriction, this diet ensures you're still getting the nutrients needed to maintain lean muscle mass, which is critical for women over 50.

How This Diet Differs from Traditional Approaches

Most diets focus on a single strategy—restricting calories, carbs, or specific food groups. The Metabolic Confusion Diet, on the other hand, is:

- **Balanced:** It doesn't eliminate any macronutrients (protein, fats, or carbs).
- **Sustainable:** The variety prevents boredom and allows for treats in moderation.
- **Effective:** It actively works to overcome the typical weight-loss plateaus that derail progress.

By alternating calorie intake, your body never "settles" into a slower metabolic state, giving you consistent results without the yo-yo effect.

Why It's Not Just Another Fad Diet

Unlike restrictive diets that feel like punishment, the Metabolic Confusion Diet is designed to fit seamlessly into your life. It's not about cutting out entire food groups or surviving on bland meals. Instead, it's about understanding your body's unique needs and nourishing it in a way that works.

Here's what makes it stand out:

- It's **realistic**: No need for elaborate meal prep or hard-to-find ingredients.
- It's **adaptable**: You can tweak the plan to fit your schedule and preferences.
- It's **empowering**: You'll feel in control of your weight loss journey, armed with a strategy that makes sense.

What You'll Gain

The Metabolic Confusion Diet isn't just about weight loss—it's about creating a healthy relationship with food, feeling confident in your body, and reclaiming your energy. By alternating high- and low-calorie days, you'll discover a system that's not only effective but also enjoyable. This isn't just another diet—it's a sustainable lifestyle tailored to your needs as an endomorph woman over 50.

Ready to reset your metabolism and finally see the results you deserve? Let's dive deeper into how this diet works and how you can make it a part of your life!

How Calorie Cycling Boosts Fat Loss and Prevents Plateaus

Weight loss plateaus are one of the most frustrating hurdles on any journey to better health. You start seeing progress, and then suddenly—it stops. The scale won't budge, your energy dips, and you're left wondering what went wrong. For endomorph women over 50, this is an especially common experience, as hormonal changes and a naturally slower metabolism can make plateaus even harder to break. This is where calorie cycling, the foundation of the Metabolic Confusion Diet, becomes a game-changer.

1. Why Do Weight Loss Plateaus Happen?

When you restrict calories for an extended period, your body begins to adapt. Your metabolism slows down to conserve energy, making it harder to burn fat. This survival mechanism is known as **metabolic adaptation** or "starvation mode." While it's a natural response, it often leaves you stuck, frustrated, and searching for solutions.

For endomorphs, this problem is compounded by:

- A predisposition to store fat more easily.
- Hormonal imbalances that make it harder to burn calories efficiently.
- A slower resting metabolic rate, even at the start of your journey.

The result? Your body stops responding to the same calorie deficit that initially worked.

2. How Calorie Cycling Works to Reset Your Metabolism

Calorie cycling involves alternating between **high-calorie days** and **low-calorie days**, which keeps your metabolism "on its toes." By consistently changing the amount of energy your body processes, you prevent it from adapting to one specific level of intake. Here's how it works:

- **High-Calorie Days**: These days give your body the energy it needs to replenish glycogen stores, fuel activity, and prevent the hormonal shifts that occur with prolonged calorie restriction. They send a signal to your metabolism that food is plentiful, keeping it active and efficient.
- **Low-Calorie Days**: These days create a calorie deficit, encouraging your body to burn stored fat for energy without triggering metabolic adaptation. By alternating these periods, your body never feels deprived for long, reducing the risk of plateaus.

Think of it as a dance between abundance and deficit: You're feeding your metabolism just enough to keep it engaged while still promoting fat loss.

3. The Hormonal Benefits of Calorie Cycling

Beyond burning calories, calorie cycling positively impacts hormones that play a key role in weight loss:

- **Leptin:** Known as the "satiety hormone," leptin tells your brain when you're full. Prolonged calorie restriction lowers leptin levels, increasing hunger and cravings. High-calorie days temporarily boost leptin levels, reducing these effects and making it easier to stick to your plan.
- **Insulin:** Endomorphs often struggle with insulin sensitivity, which can lead to fat storage and blood sugar spikes. Calorie cycling, especially when paired with nutrient-dense meals, helps regulate insulin and stabilize energy levels.
- **Cortisol:** Chronic dieting can increase cortisol (the stress hormone), which encourages fat storage, especially in the midsection. Alternating calorie levels reduces stress on your body, helping to lower cortisol levels and promote fat loss.

4. Preventing Plateaus with Strategic Variety

Calorie cycling also tackles the **boredom factor** that can sabotage traditional diets. Sticking to a low-calorie diet every day can feel restrictive and monotonous, making it harder to stay consistent. With calorie cycling, you're incorporating variety—not just in how much you eat but also in what you eat:

- **High-Calorie Days:** These can include satisfying meals with healthy carbs like sweet potatoes, whole grains, and fruits. They feel indulgent while still supporting your goals.
- **Low-Calorie Days:** These focus on lean proteins, non-starchy vegetables, and healthy fats, keeping your body in fat-burning mode.

This variety keeps both your body and mind engaged, reducing the likelihood of falling off track.

5. Real-Life Benefits for Endomorph Women Over 50

For women over 50, calorie cycling aligns perfectly with the challenges of this life stage. You'll benefit from:

- **Sustained Energy Levels:** High-calorie days provide the fuel needed for busy schedules, workouts, or simply enjoying time with family.
- **Improved Fat Loss:** By keeping your metabolism active, you'll avoid the frustrating plateaus that often come with age and hormonal changes.
- **Flexible Eating Patterns:** Calorie cycling allows for indulgences on high-calorie days, making the diet feel more sustainable long-term.

6. How This Diet Supports Long-Term Success

The beauty of calorie cycling is that it's not a short-term fix—it's a lifestyle. By alternating calorie levels, you're training your metabolism to stay responsive, making it easier to maintain your weight loss in the long run. Plus, the built-in flexibility means you can adapt the plan to fit your needs, whether you're dealing with a busy week, a vacation, or simply a craving for your favorite meal.

Key Takeaways

Calorie cycling isn't just about "tricking" your body—it's about working smarter, not harder. By alternating high- and low-calorie days, you'll avoid the metabolic slowdown that derails so many diets. Instead of fighting against your body, you'll work with it, harnessing its natural processes to burn fat, balance hormones, and feel your best. Say goodbye to plateaus and hello to steady, sustainable progress!

Chapter 3: The 5-Ingredient Recipes

Welcome to a world where cooking is simple, fast, and effective—just like the results you're aiming for with the Metabolic Confusion Diet. The 5-ingredient method isn't about cutting corners but about embracing smart, nutrient-dense combinations that fuel your body without overcomplicating your life. These recipes are crafted to balance flavor, nutrition, and convenience, using easy-to-find ingredients that won't break the bank.

Gone are the days of spending hours in the kitchen or hunting for exotic ingredients. With this approach, you'll create delicious meals in minutes—whether it's a hearty breakfast, an energizing lunch, or a satisfying dinner. Each 5-ingredient meal is thoughtfully designed to support your metabolic goals by keeping portions balanced, flavors satisfying, and prep time minimal.

This is cooking for real life—affordable, sustainable, and perfectly tailored to your journey toward better health. Let's dive in and discover how simple recipes can deliver life-changing results.

Chapter 4: High-Calorie Day Recipes
High-Calorie Breakfasts

1. Avocado and Bacon Breakfast Wrap
Preparation time: 10 minutes
Cooking time: 5 minutes
Servings: 1
Ingredients:
- 2 slices of bacon
- 1 large whole wheat tortilla
- 1/2 ripe avocado
- 1 tablespoon of salsa
- 1 egg

Instructions:
1. Cook the bacon in a skillet over medium heat until crispy, approximately 4-5 minutes. Once cooked, transfer the bacon to a paper towel-lined plate to drain and cool.
2. In the same skillet, reduce the heat to low and gently crack the egg into the skillet. Cook until the white is set but the yolk is still runny, about 3-4 minutes. If you prefer a well-done egg, flip it over and cook for an additional minute.
3. While the egg is cooking, mash the avocado in a small bowl until it reaches a smooth consistency.
4. Lay the whole wheat tortilla flat on a plate. Spread the mashed avocado evenly over the tortilla.
5. Place the cooked egg in the center of the tortilla, then add the crispy bacon on top.
6. Spoon the tablespoon of salsa over the bacon and egg.
7. Carefully fold the tortilla over the fillings, tucking in the sides as you roll, to form a wrap.
8. Serve immediately while warm.

Nutritional values: Calories: 450, Protein: 19g, Carbs: 34g, Fat: 28g, Fiber: 6g, Sodium: 720mg

2. Peanut Butter Banana Oatmeal
Preparation time: 5 minutes
Cooking time: 5 minutes
Servings: 1
Ingredients:
- 1/2 cup rolled oats
- 1 cup water or milk (for a creamier texture, use milk)
- 1 tablespoon natural peanut butter
- 1 banana, sliced
- 1 teaspoon honey (optional, for added sweetness)

Instructions:
1. In a small saucepan, bring the water or milk to a boil. Add the rolled oats and reduce the heat to a simmer. Cook for about 5 minutes, stirring occasionally, until the oats are soft and have absorbed most of the liquid.
2. Remove the saucepan from the heat. Stir in the peanut butter until it is fully incorporated into the oatmeal.
3. Add the sliced banana to the oatmeal and stir gently to combine. If you prefer your bananas slightly warmed, you can add them in step 2 with the peanut butter.
4. Transfer the oatmeal to a bowl. Drizzle with honey for added sweetness if desired.
5. Serve immediately while warm.

Nutritional values: Calories: 385, Protein: 12g, Carbs: 60g, Fat: 12g, Fiber: 7g, Sodium: 95mg

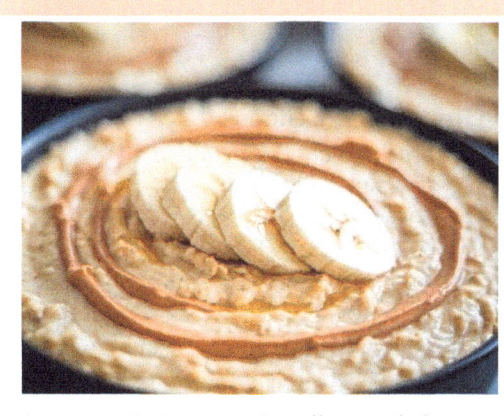

3. Ricotta and Berry Stuffed French Toast

Preparation time: 10 minutes
Cooking time: 10 minutes
Servings: 1

Ingredients:
- 2 slices of whole grain bread
- 1/2 cup of low-fat ricotta cheese
- 1/4 cup of mixed berries (blueberries, raspberries, and sliced strawberries)
- 1 tablespoon of honey
- 1 egg
- Cooking spray or a dab of butter for the pan

Instructions:
1. In a small bowl, mix the ricotta cheese with the honey until well combined.
2. Gently fold the mixed berries into the ricotta mixture, being careful not to crush the berries.
3. Spread the ricotta and berry mixture evenly over one slice of bread, leaving a small border around the edges to prevent the mixture from oozing out. Top with the second slice of bread to make a sandwich.
4. In a shallow dish, beat the egg. Dip the sandwich into the egg, ensuring both sides are well coated.
5. Heat a non-stick skillet over medium heat and coat with cooking spray or a dab of butter.
6. Place the dipped sandwich in the skillet. Cook for about 4-5 minutes on each side, or until the bread is golden brown and the filling is warm.
7. Once cooked, transfer the French toast to a plate. If desired, slice diagonally and serve warm.

Nutritional values: Calories: 350, Protein: 20g, Carbs: 45g, Fat: 10g, Fiber: 6g, Sodium: 420mg

4. Spinach and Cheese Omelette

Preparation time: 5 minutes
Cooking time: 10 minutes
Servings: 1

Ingredients:
- 2 large eggs
- 1 cup fresh spinach, chopped
- 1/4 cup shredded cheddar cheese
- 1 tablespoon olive oil
- Salt and pepper to taste

Instructions:
1. In a medium bowl, whisk the eggs until fully blended. Season with salt and pepper.
2. Heat the olive oil in a non-stick skillet over medium heat.
3. Add the chopped spinach to the skillet and sauté for 1-2 minutes, or until slightly wilted.
4. Pour the whisked eggs over the spinach. Tilt the pan to ensure the eggs evenly coat the bottom.
5. As the eggs begin to set, gently lift the edges with a spatula and tilt the pan to allow the uncooked eggs to flow to the bottom.
6. When the omelette is almost fully set, sprinkle the shredded cheddar cheese over half of the omelette.
7. Carefully fold the omelette in half, covering the cheese. Cook for another minute, or until the cheese is melted and the omelette is cooked through.
8. Transfer the omelette to a plate and serve immediately.

Nutritional values: Calories: 345, Protein: 20g, Carbs: 2g, Fat: 29g, Fiber: 1g, Sodium: 390mg

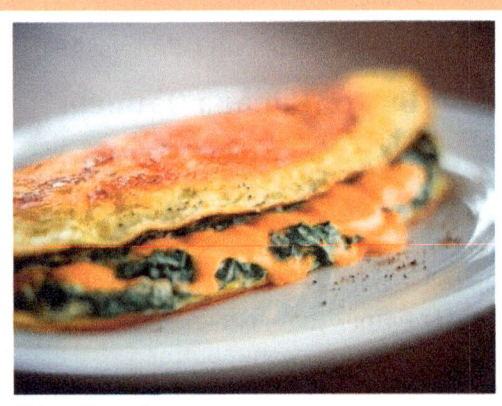

5. Smoked Salmon and Cream Cheese Bagel

Preparation time: 5 minutes
Cooking time: 0 minutes
Servings: 1 person

Ingredients:
- 1 whole grain bagel
- 2 ounces smoked salmon
- 2 tablespoons cream cheese
- 1 tablespoon capers
- 2 slices of red onion

Instructions:
1. Slice the whole grain bagel in half and toast to your preferred level of crispiness.
2. Spread 1 tablespoon of cream cheese evenly on each half of the toasted bagel.
3. Place 1 ounce of smoked salmon on top of the cream cheese on each bagel half.
4. Sprinkle 1/2 tablespoon of capers over the smoked salmon on each bagel half.
5. Add a slice of red onion on top of the capers for a crisp, flavorful finish.
6. Serve immediately and enjoy a balanced, high-calorie breakfast that supports your metabolic confusion diet.

Nutritional values: Calories: 400, Protein: 23g, Carbs: 44g, Fat: 16g, Fiber: 6g, Sodium: 1200mg

6. Almond Butter and Honey Pancakes

Preparation time: 10 minutes
Cooking time: 15 minutes
Servings: 1

Ingredients:
- 1/2 cup almond flour
- 1 large egg
- 2 tablespoons almond butter
- 1 tablespoon honey, plus more for drizzling
- 1/4 teaspoon baking powder

Instructions:
1. In a medium mixing bowl, whisk together the almond flour and baking powder.
2. Add the egg, almond butter, and honey to the bowl. Stir until all ingredients are well combined and a batter forms. If the batter is too thick, add a teaspoon of water to reach the desired consistency.
3. Heat a non-stick skillet over medium heat. Once hot, pour 1/4 cup of the batter onto the skillet to form a pancake. Cook for about 2-3 minutes, or until bubbles form on the surface and the edges appear set.
4. Carefully flip the pancake and cook for an additional 2-3 minutes, or until golden brown and cooked through.
5. Repeat with the remaining batter, making sure to stir the batter before pouring each pancake.
6. Serve the pancakes warm, drizzled with additional honey if desired.

Nutritional values: Calories: 485, Protein: 14g, Carbs: 34g, Fat: 35g, Fiber: 6g, Sodium: 136mg

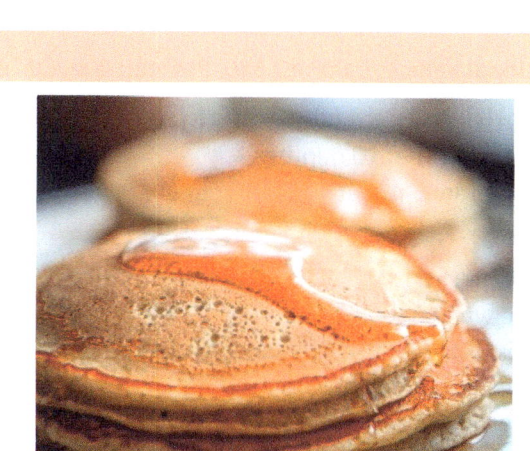

7. Sausage and Egg Breakfast Bowl

Preparation time: 10 minutes
Cooking time: 15 minutes
Servings: 1

Ingredients:
- 2 large eggs
- 1/4 pound turkey sausage
- 1/2 cup cooked quinoa
- 1/4 cup shredded cheddar cheese
- 1 tablespoon olive oil

Instructions:
1. Heat the olive oil in a skillet over medium heat. Add the turkey sausage, breaking it apart with a spatula, and cook until browned and no longer pink, about 5-7 minutes. Remove from skillet and set aside.
2. In the same skillet, reduce heat to low and gently crack the eggs into the skillet. Cook to your desired level of doneness, about 3-4 minutes for soft yolks.
3. While the eggs are cooking, place the cooked quinoa in a microwave-safe bowl and heat for 45 seconds, or until warm.
4. Assemble the breakfast bowl by placing the warm quinoa at the bottom. Top with the cooked turkey sausage.
5. Carefully place the cooked eggs over the sausage and sprinkle the shredded cheddar cheese on top.
6. Serve immediately while warm.

Nutritional values: Calories: 580, Protein: 40g, Carbs: 32g, Fat: 32g, Fiber: 3g, Sodium: 870mg

8. Cheddar and Ham Breakfast Quesadilla

Preparation time: 10 minutes
Cooking time: 5 minutes
Servings: 1

Ingredients:
- 1 large whole wheat tortilla
- 2 slices of ham, roughly chopped
- 1/2 cup shredded cheddar cheese
- 1 tablespoon olive oil
- 1/4 cup diced tomatoes (optional for added freshness)

Instructions:
1. Heat a non-stick skillet over medium heat and add the olive oil.
2. Place the whole wheat tortilla in the skillet, ensuring it's evenly coated with olive oil.
3. On one half of the tortilla, evenly distribute the chopped ham.
4. Sprinkle the shredded cheddar cheese over the ham.
5. If using, add the diced tomatoes on top of the cheese.
6. Fold the other half of the tortilla over the filling to create a half-moon shape.
7. Cook for about 2 minutes, then carefully flip the quesadilla with a spatula to brown the other side, allowing another 2-3 minutes for the cheese to melt fully.
8. Once both sides are golden brown and the cheese is melted, transfer the quesadilla to a cutting board.
9. Cut the quesadilla into wedges and serve immediately.

Nutritional values: Calories: 450, Protein: 28g, Carbs: 35g, Fat: 23g, Fiber: 5g, Sodium: 890mg

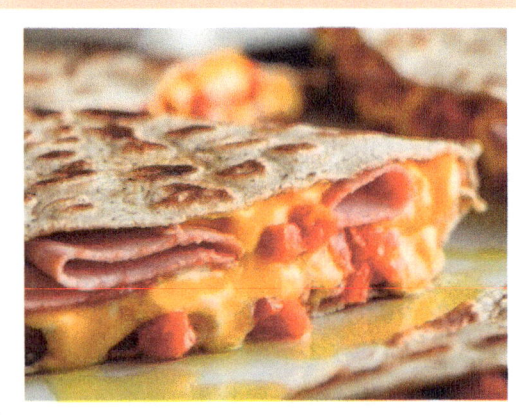

9. Greek Yogurt and Granola Parfait

Preparation time: 5 minutes
Cooking time: 0 minutes
Servings: 1

Ingredients:
- 1 cup Greek yogurt, full-fat
- 1/2 cup granola, preferably with nuts and dried fruits
- 1 tablespoon honey
- 1/2 cup mixed berries (strawberries, blueberries, raspberries)
- 1 tablespoon almond slices

Instructions:
1. In a glass or bowl, layer half of the Greek yogurt at the bottom.
2. Add a layer of 1/4 cup granola over the yogurt.
3. Drizzle half of the honey over the granola.
4. Add a layer of mixed berries on top of the granola.
5. Add another layer with the remaining Greek yogurt.
6. Top with the remaining 1/4 cup granola and the remaining honey.
7. Garnish with almond slices.
8. Serve immediately for the best texture or refrigerate for up to an hour before serving to allow the flavors to meld.

Nutritional values: Calories: 450, Protein: 25g, Carbs: 55g, Fat: 18g, Fiber: 6g, Sodium: 105mg

10. Mushroom and Swiss Cheese Frittata

Preparation time: 10 minutes
Cooking time: 20 minutes
Servings: 1

Ingredients:
- 4 large eggs
- 1 cup sliced mushrooms
- 1/4 cup shredded Swiss cheese
- 1 tablespoon olive oil
- Salt and pepper to taste

Instructions:
1. Preheat your oven to 375°F (190°C).
2. In a medium bowl, whisk the eggs until fully blended. Season with salt and pepper.
3. Heat olive oil in an oven-safe skillet over medium heat. Add the sliced mushrooms and sauté until they are soft and browned, about 5 minutes.
4. Pour the beaten eggs over the mushrooms in the skillet. Tilt the skillet to ensure the eggs evenly cover all the mushrooms.
5. Sprinkle the shredded Swiss cheese on top of the egg and mushroom mixture.
6. Transfer the skillet to the preheated oven. Bake until the eggs are set and the cheese is melted and slightly golden, about 15 minutes.
7. Carefully remove the skillet from the oven (the handle will be hot) and let the frittata cool for a couple of minutes.
8. Slide the frittata onto a plate, slice, and serve.

Nutritional values: Calories: 400, Protein: 28g, Carbs: 6g, Fat: 30g, Fiber: 1g, Sodium: 340mg

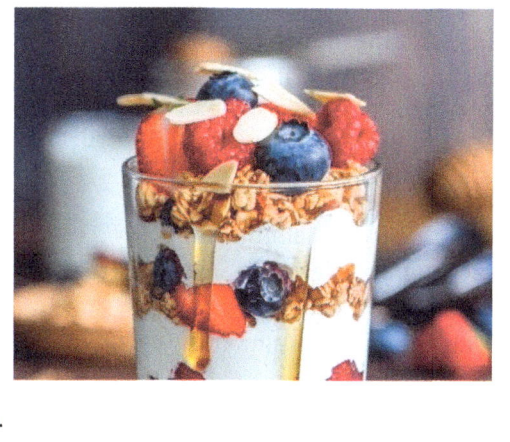

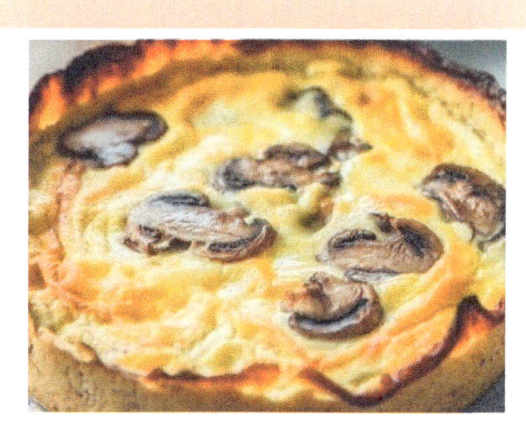

11. Chia Seed Pudding with Mixed Nuts

Preparation time: 5 minutes
Resting time: 4 hours or overnight
Servings: 1

Ingredients:
- 1/4 cup chia seeds
- 1 cup unsweetened almond milk
- 1 tablespoon maple syrup
- 1/4 teaspoon vanilla extract
- 1/4 cup mixed nuts (almonds, walnuts, and pecans), roughly chopped

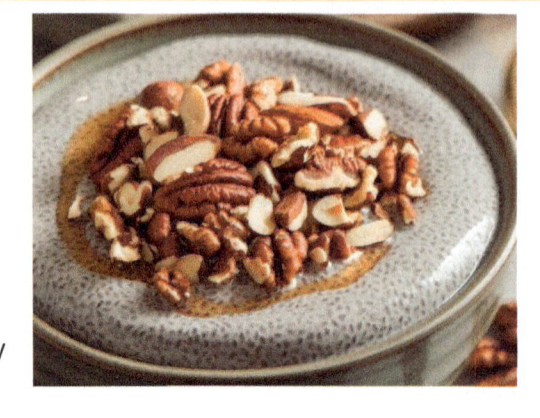

Instructions:
1. In a medium-sized bowl, combine the chia seeds, almond milk, maple syrup, and vanilla extract. Stir well until all the ingredients are fully mixed.
2. Cover the bowl with a lid or plastic wrap. Refrigerate for at least 4 hours, preferably overnight, until the mixture reaches a pudding-like consistency.
3. Once the chia pudding has set, give it a good stir to break up any clumps. If the pudding is too thick, you can add a little more almond milk to reach your desired consistency.
4. Top the pudding with the mixed nuts just before serving.

Nutritional values: Calories: 345, Protein: 10g, Carbs: 34g, Fat: 20g, Fiber: 15g, Sodium: 180mg

12. Turkey and Avocado Breakfast Sandwich

Preparation time: 10 minutes
Cooking time: 5 minutes
Servings: 1

Ingredients:
- 2 slices of whole-grain bread
- 3 ounces of sliced turkey breast
- 1/2 ripe avocado
- 1 tablespoon of mayonnaise
- 1 leaf of lettuce

Instructions:
1. Toast the whole-grain bread slices to your desired level of crispiness.
2. While the bread is toasting, slice the avocado thinly.
3. Spread the mayonnaise evenly over one side of each slice of toasted bread.
4. On one slice of bread, layer the sliced turkey breast on top of the mayonnaise.
5. Add the sliced avocado on top of the turkey slices.
6. Place the lettuce leaf on top of the avocado.
7. Cover with the second slice of bread, mayonnaise side down, to complete the sandwich.
8. If preferred, cut the sandwich in half for easier eating.

Nutritional values: Calories: 450, Protein: 25g, Carbs: 35g, Fat: 23g, Fiber: 7g, Sodium: 720mg

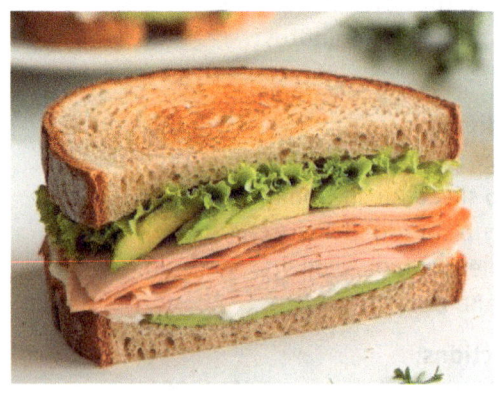

High-Calorie Lunch Recipes

13. Grilled Chicken and Avocado Salad

Preparation time: 10 minutes
Cooking time: 10 minutes
Servings: 1

Ingredients:
- 6 oz chicken breast
- 1 ripe avocado, sliced
- 2 cups mixed greens (e.g., spinach, arugula, and romaine)
- 1 tablespoon olive oil
- 1 tablespoon balsamic vinegar

Instructions:
1. Preheat your grill to medium-high heat. While the grill is heating, brush the chicken breast with half of the olive oil and season with salt and pepper to taste.
2. Grill the chicken for 5 minutes per side, or until it reaches 165°F and juices run clear. Let rest, then slice into strips.
3. In a large bowl, toss the mixed greens with the remaining olive oil and balsamic vinegar.
4. Add the sliced avocado to the greens.
5. Top the salad with the grilled chicken strips.
6. Serve immediately, enjoying the blend of flavors and textures from the creamy avocado, tangy balsamic, and hearty grilled chicken.

Nutritional values: Calories: 600, Protein: 38g, Carbs: 18g, Fat: 44g, Fiber: 8g, Sodium: 200mg

14. Quinoa and Black Bean Burrito Bowl

Preparation time: 15 minutes
Cooking time: 20 minutes
Servings: 1

Ingredients:
- 1/2 cup quinoa, rinsed
- 1 cup water
- 1/2 cup black beans, drained and rinsed
- 1/2 cup corn kernels, fresh or frozen
- 1/4 cup salsa
- 1/4 cup shredded cheddar cheese

Instructions:
1. In a small saucepan, boil 1 cup of water. Add quinoa, reduce heat to low, cover, and simmer for 15-20 minutes until tender and water is absorbed. Let sit for 5 minutes, then fluff with a fork.
2. While the quinoa is cooking, drain and rinse canned black beans. If using frozen corn, thaw it at room temperature or in the microwave.
3. In a microwave-safe bowl, combine quinoa, black beans, and corn. Microwave for 1-2 minutes until heated.
4. Stir in the salsa until everything is well combined and evenly coated.
5. Transfer the mixture to a serving bowl and top with shredded cheddar cheese..
6. Microwave the bowl for an additional 30-60 seconds, or until the cheese is melted.
7. Serve the burrito bowl hot as a nourishing, high-calorie lunch option.

Nutritional values: Calories: 540, Protein: 22g, Carbs: 92g, Fat: 12g, Fiber: 15g, Sodium: 690mg

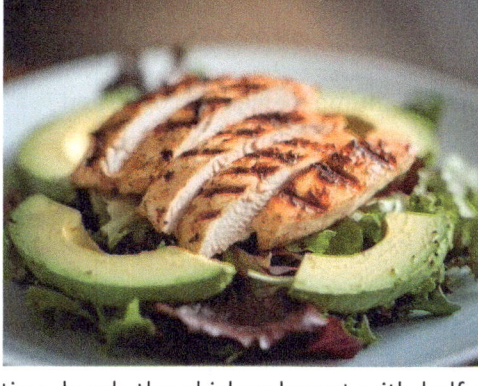

15. Shrimp and Spinach Stir-Fry

Preparation time: 10 minutes
Cooking time: 10 minutes
Servings: 1
Ingredients:
- 4 ounces of shrimp, peeled and deveined
- 2 cups of fresh spinach
- 1 tablespoon of olive oil
- 1 teaspoon of minced garlic
- 1/4 teaspoon of red pepper flakes (optional for added heat)

Instructions:
1. Heat the olive oil in a large skillet over medium heat.
2. Add the minced garlic and red pepper flakes to the skillet, sautéing for about 1 minute until the garlic is fragrant but not browned.
3. Increase the heat to medium-high and add the shrimp to the skillet. Cook for 2-3 minutes on one side until they start to turn pink.
4. Flip the shrimp and cook for an additional 2 minutes, or until they are fully pink and cooked through.
5. Reduce the heat to medium. Add the fresh spinach to the skillet, stirring frequently, until the spinach wilts and reduces in volume, about 2-3 minutes.
6. Once the spinach is wilted, stir the shrimp and spinach together to combine the flavors. Cook for an additional minute to ensure everything is heated through.
7. Remove the skillet from the heat and transfer the shrimp and spinach stir-fry to a plate.

Nutritional values: Calories: 295, Protein: 24g, Carbs: 4g, Fat: 20g, Fiber: 1g, Sodium: 560mg

16. Beef and Broccoli Power Bowl

Preparation time: 15 minutes
Cooking time: 10 minutes
Servings: 1

Ingredients:
- 1/2 pound beef sirloin, thinly sliced
- 2 cups broccoli florets
- 1 tablespoon olive oil
- 2 tablespoons soy sauce (low sodium)
- 1 tablespoon honey

Instructions:
1. Heat the olive oil in a large skillet over medium-high heat. Add the beef sirloin slices and stir-fry for about 3-4 minutes, or until they are browned and nearly cooked through. Remove the beef from the skillet and set aside.
2. In the same skillet, add the broccoli florets. Stir-fry for about 2-3 minutes, or until the broccoli is vibrant and tender-crisp.
3. Return the beef to the skillet with the broccoli. Reduce the heat to medium.
4. In a small bowl, whisk together the soy sauce and honey until well combined. Pour this mixture over the beef and broccoli in the skillet. Stir well to ensure the beef and broccoli are evenly coated with the sauce.
5. Continue to cook for another 2-3 minutes, stirring frequently, until the sauce has thickened slightly and everything is heated through.
6. Serve the beef and broccoli power bowl immediately.

Nutritional values: Calories: 600, Protein: 55g, Carbs: 35g, Fat: 25g, Fiber: 5g, Sodium: 800mg

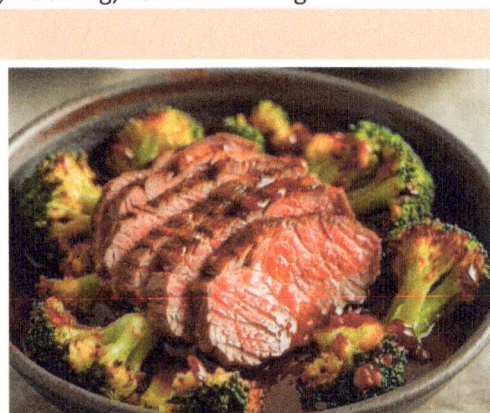

17. Turkey and Sweet Potato Skillet

Preparation time: 15 minutes
Cooking time: 20 minutes
Servings: 1

Ingredients:
- 1/2 pound sweet potatoes, peeled and diced
- 4 ounces turkey breast, cut into cubes
- 1 tablespoon olive oil
- 1/4 teaspoon salt
- 1/4 teaspoon black pepper

Instructions:
1. Heat the olive oil in a large skillet over medium heat. Add the diced sweet potatoes to the skillet and season with salt and pepper. Cook for about 10 minutes, stirring occasionally, until the sweet potatoes are slightly softened.
2. Add the cubed turkey breast to the skillet with the sweet potatoes. Stir to combine and cook for an additional 10 minutes, or until the turkey is cooked through and the sweet potatoes are tender.
3. Once the turkey is fully cooked and the sweet potatoes are fork-tender, increase the heat to medium-high for 2-3 minutes to add a slight crisp to the outside of the sweet potatoes, stirring frequently to prevent burning.
4. Remove the skillet from the heat and let it sit for a minute before serving to allow the flavors to meld together.

Nutritional values: Calories: 420, Protein: 26g, Carbs: 45g, Fat: 15g, Fiber: 7g, Sodium: 320mg

18. Chicken and Quinoa Stuffed Peppers

Preparation time: 15 minutes
Cooking time: 30 minutes
Servings: 1
Ingredients:
- 2 bell peppers, halved and seeded
- 1/2 cup cooked quinoa
- 1/4 pound chicken breast, cooked and shredded
- 1/4 cup shredded mozzarella cheese
- 1 tablespoon olive oil

Instructions:
1. Preheat your oven to 375°F (190°C).
2. Place the bell pepper halves on a baking sheet, cut side up. Drizzle with olive oil.
3. In a mixing bowl, combine the cooked quinoa and shredded chicken breast. Mix well.
4. Spoon the quinoa and chicken mixture evenly into the bell pepper halves.
5. Sprinkle the shredded mozzarella cheese over the top of each stuffed pepper.
6. Bake in the preheated oven for about 25-30 minutes, or until the peppers are tender and the cheese is bubbly and slightly golden.
7. Remove from the oven and let cool for a couple of minutes before serving.

Nutritional values: Calories: 560, Protein: 38g, Carbs: 44g, Fat: 26g, Fiber: 8g, Sodium: 320mg

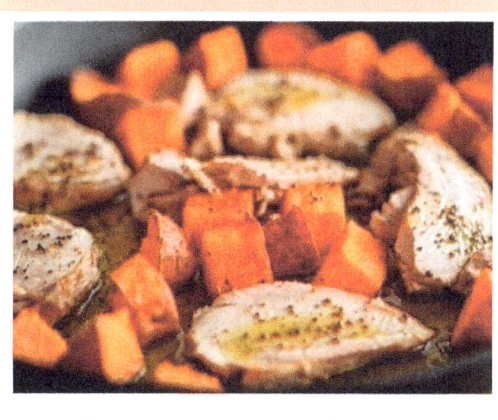

19. Lentil and Kale Soup

Preparation time: 10 minutes
Cooking time: 25 minutes
Servings: 1

Ingredients:
- 1/2 cup dried lentils, rinsed
- 2 cups low-sodium vegetable broth
- 1 cup kale, chopped
- 1/2 teaspoon garlic powder
- 1/2 teaspoon onion powder

Instructions:
1. In a medium-sized pot, combine the rinsed lentils and low-sodium vegetable broth. Bring the mixture to a boil over high heat.
2. Once boiling, reduce the heat to low, cover, and simmer for 20 minutes, or until the lentils are tender.
3. Add the chopped kale, garlic powder, and onion powder to the pot. Stir well to combine.
4. Continue to simmer for an additional 5 minutes, or until the kale is wilted and tender.
5. Taste and adjust the seasoning if necessary. If the soup is too thick, add a little more vegetable broth or water to reach your desired consistency.
6. Serve the soup hot.

Nutritional values: Calories: 310, Protein: 19g, Carbs: 54g, Fat: 1g, Fiber: 15g, Sodium: 120mg

20. Tuna and White Bean Salad

Preparation time: 10 minutes
Cooking time: 0 minutes
Servings: 1

Ingredients:
- 1 can (5 ounces) tuna in water, drained
- 1 can (15 ounces) white beans, rinsed and drained
- 1 tablespoon olive oil
- 2 tablespoons red onion, finely chopped
- Salt and pepper to taste

Instructions:
1. In a medium bowl, combine the drained tuna and rinsed white beans.
2. Add the finely chopped red onion to the bowl.
3. Drizzle the olive oil over the tuna, beans, and onion.
4. Season with salt and pepper to taste.
5. Gently mix all the ingredients until well combined, being careful not to mash the beans.
6. Taste and adjust the seasoning if necessary.
7. Serve immediately or chill in the refrigerator for 30 minutes before serving if you prefer a colder salad.

Nutritional values: Calories: 485, Protein: 42g, Carbs: 53g, Fat: 14g, Fiber: 13g, Sodium: 595mg

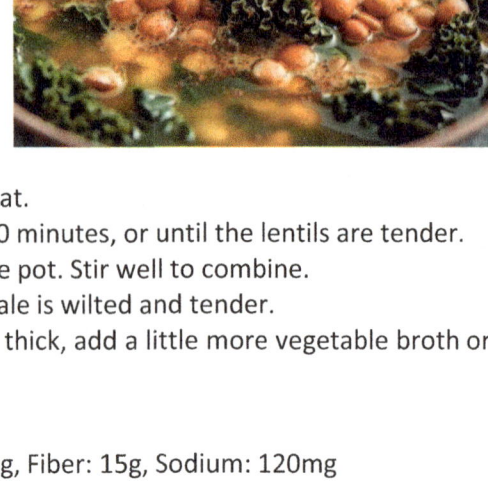

21. Steak and Arugula Wrap

Preparation time: 10 minutes
Cooking time: 6 minutes
Servings: 1

Ingredients:
- 4 oz sirloin steak
- 1 cup arugula
- 1 large whole wheat tortilla
- 2 tablespoons blue cheese, crumbled
- 1 tablespoon balsamic glaze

Instructions:
1. Preheat a grill pan or skillet over medium-high heat. Season the sirloin steak with salt and pepper to taste. Place the steak on the grill pan and cook for about 3 minutes on each side for medium-rare, or until it reaches your desired level of doneness. Remove the steak from the grill and let it rest for a few minutes.
2. While the steak is resting, warm the whole wheat tortilla in a dry skillet over medium heat for about 30 seconds on each side, or until it's pliable and slightly toasted.
3. Thinly slice the rested steak against the grain to make it easier to eat in the wrap.
4. Lay the warm tortilla flat on a plate. Arrange the arugula in the center of the tortilla, leaving space at the edges for folding.
5. Place the sliced steak on top of the arugula. Sprinkle the crumbled blue cheese over the steak.
6. Drizzle the balsamic glaze over the steak and cheese.
7. Fold the sides of the tortilla in, then roll it up tightly from the bottom to enclose the filling.
8. Cut the wrap in half diagonally and serve immediately.

Nutritional values: Calories: 490, Protein: 38g, Carbs: 35g, Fat: 22g, Fiber: 4g, Sodium: 620mg

22. Sesame Ginger Salmon Bowl

Preparation time: 15 minutes
Cooking time: 15 minutes
Servings: 1

Ingredients:
- 1 salmon fillet (about 6 ounces)
- 1 tablespoon sesame oil
- 1 tablespoon soy sauce (low sodium)
- 1 teaspoon fresh ginger, grated
- 1 cup cooked brown rice
- 1/4 cup green onions, sliced for garnish

Instructions:
1. Preheat your oven to 400°F (200°C). Line a baking sheet with aluminum foil for easy cleanup.
2. In a small bowl, whisk together the sesame oil, soy sauce, and grated ginger to create the marinade.
3. Place the salmon fillet on the prepared baking sheet. Brush the salmon generously with the marinade, ensuring both sides are coated.
4. Bake the salmon in the preheated oven for 12-15 minutes, or until the salmon flakes easily with a fork.
5. While the salmon is baking, prepare 1 cup of cooked brown rice according to package instructions.
6. Once the salmon is done, remove it from the oven and let it rest for a couple of minutes.
7. Place the cooked brown rice in a bowl. Top with the baked salmon fillet.
8. Garnish the salmon bowl with sliced green onions.
9. Serve immediately while warm.

Nutritional values: Calories: 620, Protein: 36g, Carbs: 45g, Fat: 32g, Fiber: 4g, Sodium: 620mg

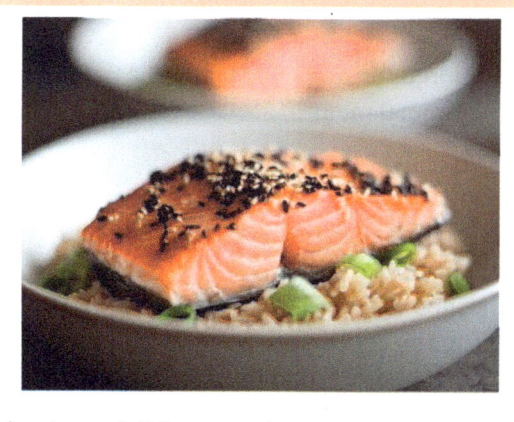

23. Chicken and Zucchini Noodles

Preparation time: 10 minutes
Cooking time: 15 minutes
Servings: 1

Ingredients:
- 1 large chicken breast (about 6 ounces)
- 2 medium zucchinis
- 1 tablespoon olive oil
- 1/4 cup grated Parmesan cheese
- Salt and pepper to taste

Instructions:
1. Season the chicken breast with salt and pepper. In a skillet over medium heat, heat the olive oil. Add the chicken breast and cook for about 6-7 minutes on each side, or until fully cooked and no longer pink in the center. Remove from the skillet and let it rest for a few minutes before slicing it thinly.
2. While the chicken is resting, use a spiralizer to turn the zucchinis into noodles. If you don't have a spiralizer, you can use a vegetable peeler to create thin zucchini ribbons.
3. In the same skillet used for the chicken, add the zucchini noodles. Sauté for about 2-3 minutes, just until the noodles are tender. Avoid overcooking to prevent the noodles from becoming too soft.
4. Add the sliced chicken to the skillet with the zucchini noodles, tossing gently to combine. Cook for an additional 2 minutes to ensure everything is heated through.
5. Serve the chicken and zucchini noodles hot, sprinkled with grated Parmesan cheese.

Nutritional values: Calories: 450, Protein: 55g, Carbs: 10g, Fat: 20g, Fiber: 3g, Sodium: 320mg

24. Pork and Apple Slaw

Preparation time: 15 minutes
Cooking time: 0 minutes
Servings: 1

Ingredients:
- 1 cup shredded cooked pork loin
- 1 medium apple, julienned
- 1 tablespoon olive oil
- 1 tablespoon apple cider vinegar
- Salt and pepper to taste

Instructions:
1. In a large mixing bowl, combine the shredded cooked pork loin and julienned apple.
2. Drizzle the olive oil and apple cider vinegar over the pork and apple mixture.
3. Season with salt and pepper to taste.
4. Toss everything together until the pork and apple are well coated with the dressing.
5. Let the slaw sit for about 10 minutes to allow the flavors to meld together.
6. Serve the pork and apple slaw chilled or at room temperature.

Nutritional values: Calories: 320, Protein: 22g, Carbs: 15g, Fat: 18g, Fiber: 3g, Sodium: 65mg

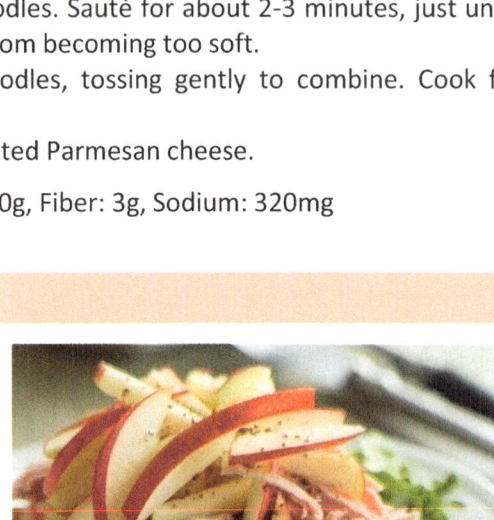

25. Balsamic Mushroom and Spinach Pasta

Preparation time: 15 minutes
Cooking time: 20 minutes
Servings: 1

Ingredients:
- 2 ounces whole wheat pasta
- 1 cup fresh spinach
- 1/2 cup sliced mushrooms
- 2 tablespoons balsamic vinegar
- 1 tablespoon olive oil

Instructions:
1. Bring a large pot of salted water to a boil. Add the whole wheat pasta and cook according to package instructions until al dente, about 8-10 minutes. Drain and set aside.
2. While the pasta is cooking, heat the olive oil in a large skillet over medium heat. Add the sliced mushrooms and sauté until they are soft and lightly browned, about 5-7 minutes.
3. Add the spinach to the skillet with the mushrooms. Cook, stirring occasionally, until the spinach has wilted, about 2-3 minutes.
4. Pour the balsamic vinegar into the skillet with the mushrooms and spinach. Stir well to combine and cook for an additional 2 minutes, allowing the flavors to meld together.
5. Add the cooked pasta to the skillet with the mushroom and spinach mixture. Toss everything together to ensure the pasta is evenly coated with the balsamic sauce.
6. Serve the pasta hot, directly from the skillet.

Nutritional values: Calories: 420, Protein: 14g, Carbs: 68g, Fat: 12g, Fiber: 10g, Sodium: 95mg

26. Spicy Chickpea and Tomato Stew

Preparation time: 10 minutes
Cooking time: 25 minutes
Servings: 1

Ingredients:
- 1/2 cup canned chickpeas, drained and rinsed
- 1 cup diced tomatoes (fresh or canned)
- 1/2 teaspoon cumin
- 1/4 teaspoon red pepper flakes (adjust to taste)
- 1 tablespoon olive oil

Instructions:
1. Heat the olive oil in a medium saucepan over medium heat. Add the cumin and red pepper flakes, stirring for about 1 minute until fragrant.
2. Add the diced tomatoes to the saucepan, including juices if using canned. Bring to a simmer.
3. Stir in the chickpeas and continue to simmer for about 20-25 minutes, or until the stew has thickened to your liking.
4. Taste and adjust the seasoning, adding more red pepper flakes if you prefer a spicier stew.
5. Serve hot. This stew can be enjoyed on its own or paired with a side of whole grain bread for dipping.

Nutritional values: Calories: 295, Protein: 9g, Carbs: 35g, Fat: 14g, Fiber: 9g, Sodium: 300mg

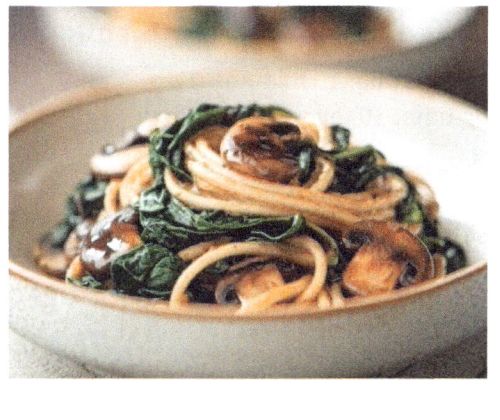

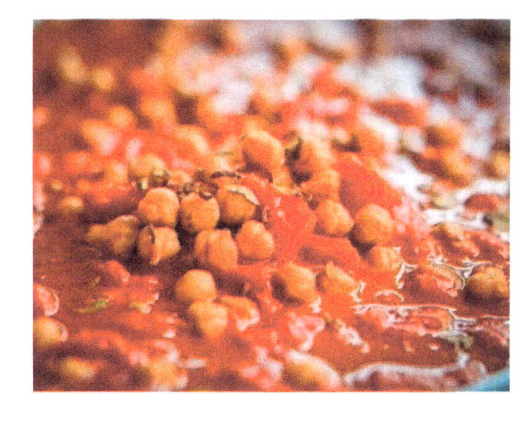

High-Calorie Dinners

27. Grilled Steak with Chimichurri Sauce

Preparation time: 15 minutes
Cooking time: 10 minutes
Servings: 1

Ingredients:
- 6 oz sirloin steak
- 1/2 cup fresh parsley
- 2 cloves garlic, minced
- 2 tablespoons olive oil
- 1 tablespoon red wine vinegar

Instructions:
1. Preheat your grill to medium-high heat. While the grill is heating, let the steak rest at room temperature for about 10 minutes, to ensure even cooking.
2. For the chimichurri sauce, finely chop parsley and place it in a small bowl. Add garlic, olive oil, and red wine vinegar, then stir to combine. Set aside.
3. Season the sirloin steak on both sides with salt and pepper to taste. Place the steak on the hot grill.
4. Grill the steak for 4-5 minutes per side for medium-rare, or adjust time based on your preferred doneness.
5. Once cooked, remove the steak and let it rest for 5 minutes to lock in the juices.
6. After resting, slice the steak thinly against the grain for tenderness.
7. Serve the sliced steak with a generous spoonful of the chimichurri sauce drizzled over the top.

Nutritional values: Calories: 540, Protein: 46g, Carbs: 2g, Fat: 38g, Fiber: 0.5g, Sodium: 120mg

28. Creamy Shrimp Alfredo with Spinach

Preparation time: 15 minutes
Cooking time: 15 minutes
Servings: 1

Ingredients:
- 4 oz fettuccine pasta
- 4 oz shrimp, peeled and deveined
- 1 cup fresh spinach
- 1/4 cup light Alfredo sauce
- 1 tablespoon olive oil

Instructions:
1. Bring a large pot of salted water to a boil. Cook the fettuccine according to package instructions (about 8-10 minutes). Drain and set aside.
2. While the pasta is cooking, heat olive oil in a skillet over medium heat. Cook the shrimp for 2-3 minutes per side, until pink and opaque. Remove and set aside.
3. In the same skillet, sauté spinach for 1-2 minutes until wilted. Remove from heat.
4. Return the cooked shrimp to the skillet with the spinach. Add the cooked fettuccine pasta and light Alfredo sauce. Gently toss to combine over low heat, ensuring the pasta is evenly coated with the sauce and the ingredients are well mixed.
5. Once everything is heated through and well combined, about 2-3 minutes, remove from heat.
6. Serve the creamy shrimp Alfredo with spinach hot.

Nutritional values: Calories: 580, Protein: 35g, Carbs: 58g, Fat: 22g, Fiber: 3g, Sodium: 610mg

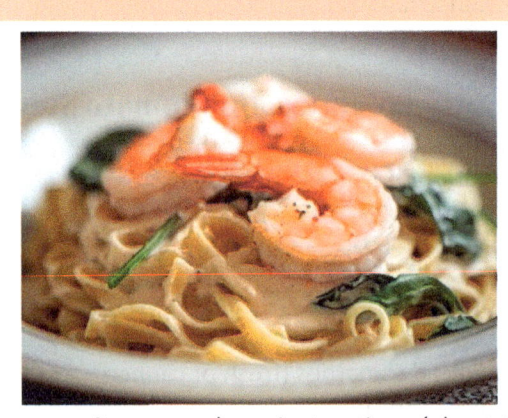

29. Honey Garlic Pork Chops

Preparation time: 5 minutes
Cooking time: 12 minutes
Servings: 1
Ingredients:
- 1 (6-ounce) pork chop, about 1-inch thick
- 2 tablespoons honey
- 1 tablespoon soy sauce (low sodium)
- 2 cloves garlic, minced
- 1 tablespoon olive oil

Instructions:
1. In a small bowl, whisk together the honey, soy sauce, and minced garlic to create the marinade.
2. Place the pork chop in a dish and pour the marinade over it, coating both sides. Let it marinate for 15 minutes at room temperature or up to 2 hours in the fridge.
3. Heat the olive oil in a skillet over medium-high heat. Once hot, add the marinated pork chop to the skillet, reserving the excess marinade.
4. Cook the pork chop for about 5-6 minutes on one side, then flip and cook for an additional 5-6 minutes on the other side, or until the internal temperature reaches 145°F (63°C).
5. While the pork chop is cooking, pour the reserved marinade into a small saucepan and bring to a boil over medium heat. Reduce the heat and simmer for 2-3 minutes, or until the sauce thickens slightly.
6. Once the pork chop is cooked, transfer it to a plate and let it rest for 3 minutes.
7. Drizzle the thickened sauce over the pork chop before serving.

Nutritional values: Calories: 495, Protein: 35g, Carbs: 35g, Fat: 23g, Fiber: 0g, Sodium: 510mg

30. Chicken Alfredo with Broccoli

Preparation time: 15 minutes
Cooking time: 20 minutes
Servings: 1
Ingredients:
- 6 oz chicken breast, cut into bite-sized pieces
- 1 cup broccoli florets
- 1/2 cup heavy cream
- 1/4 cup grated Parmesan cheese
- 1 tablespoon olive oil

Instructions:
1. Heat the olive oil in a large skillet over medium heat. Add the chicken pieces and cook until they are golden brown and cooked through, about 6-8 minutes. Remove the chicken from the skillet and set aside.
2. In the same skillet, add the broccoli florets and sauté for about 3-4 minutes, or until they are bright green and slightly tender. You may add a splash of water to help steam the broccoli.
3. Lower the heat and add the heavy cream to the skillet with the broccoli. Stir well to combine.
4. Add the grated Parmesan cheese to the skillet, stirring continuously, until the cheese has melted into the cream and the sauce has thickened slightly, about 2-3 minutes.
5. Return the cooked chicken to the skillet. Stir well to ensure the chicken is coated in the Alfredo sauce and heated through.
6. Serve the Chicken Alfredo with Broccoli hot, ensuring a balanced distribution of chicken, broccoli, and sauce in each serving.

Nutritional values: Calories: 785, Protein: 58g, Carbs: 9g, Fat: 58g, Fiber: 2g, Sodium: 540mg

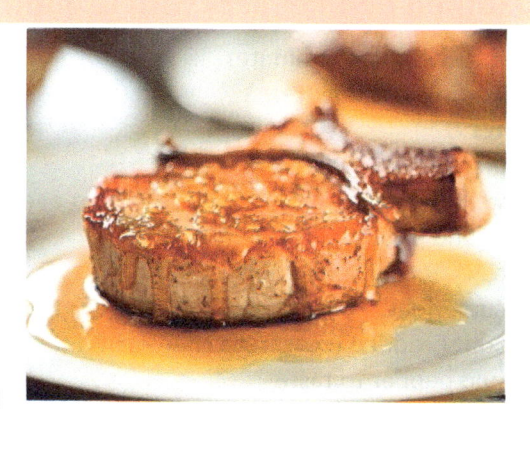

31. Stuffed Bell Peppers with Ground Beef

Preparation time: 15 minutes
Cooking time: 45 minutes
Servings: 1
Ingredients:
- 2 large bell peppers, halved and seeds removed
- 1/2 pound ground beef
- 1/2 cup cooked brown rice
- 1/4 cup tomato sauce
- 1/4 cup shredded mozzarella cheese
- Salt and pepper to taste

Instructions:
1. Preheat your oven to 375°F (190°C).
2. In a skillet over medium heat, cook the ground beef until it's no longer pink, breaking it apart with a spoon as it cooks. Season with salt and pepper.
3. Combine the cooked ground beef, cooked brown rice, and tomato sauce in a bowl. Mix well.
4. Arrange the bell pepper halves in a baking dish, cut side up.
5. Spoon the beef and rice mixture into each bell pepper half, pressing down slightly to pack the mixture in.
6. Cover the baking dish with aluminum foil and bake in the preheated oven for 35 minutes.
7. Remove the foil, sprinkle the shredded mozzarella cheese over each stuffed pepper, and return to the oven, uncovered, for an additional 10 minutes, or until the cheese is melted and bubbly.
8. Let the stuffed bell peppers cool for a few minutes before serving.

Nutritional values: Calories: 600, Protein: 36g, Carbs: 48g, Fat: 30g, Fiber: 6g, Sodium: 700mg

32. Maple Glazed Salmon with Quinoa

Preparation time: 15 minutes
Cooking time: 20 minutes
Servings: 1

Ingredients:
- 1 salmon fillet (about 6 ounces)
- 1/2 cup quinoa
- 1 tablespoon maple syrup
- 1 tablespoon soy sauce (low sodium)
- 1 tablespoon olive oil

Instructions:
1. Rinse the quinoa under cold water until the water runs clear. In a small saucepan, combine the quinoa with 1 cup of water. Bring to a boil, then reduce heat to low, cover, and simmer for 15 minutes, or until all the water is absorbed. Remove from heat and let it stand for 5 minutes, then fluff with a fork.
2. Preheat the oven to 400°F (200°C). Line a baking sheet with aluminum foil and lightly grease it with olive oil.
3. In a small bowl, mix together the maple syrup and soy sauce. Place the salmon fillet on the prepared baking sheet and brush it with the maple syrup and soy sauce mixture, ensuring it's evenly coated.
4. Bake the salmon in the preheated oven for about 12-15 minutes, or until the fish flakes easily with a fork.
5. Serve the baked salmon over a bed of fluffy quinoa.

Nutritional values: Calories: 560, Protein: 38g, Carbs: 55g, Fat: 22g, Fiber: 5g, Sodium: 530mg

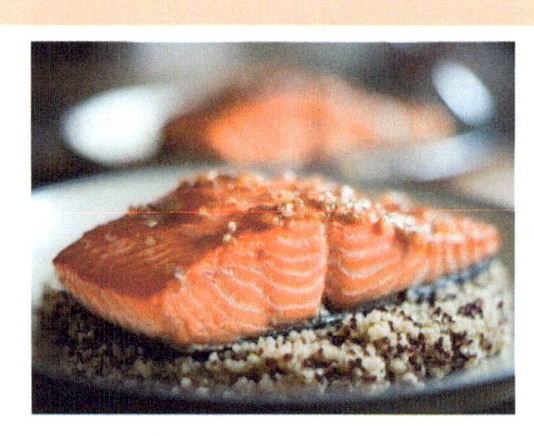

33. Beef Stroganoff with Mushrooms

Preparation time: 15 minutes
Cooking time: 20 minutes
Servings: 1

Ingredients:
- 1/2 pound lean beef sirloin, thinly sliced
- 1 cup sliced mushrooms
- 1/2 cup beef broth (low sodium)
- 1/4 cup sour cream (light)
- 1 tablespoon olive oil

Instructions:
1. Heat the olive oil in a large skillet over medium-high heat. Add the sliced beef sirloin to the skillet and cook for about 3-4 minutes, or until browned. Remove the beef from the skillet and set aside.
2. In the same skillet, add the sliced mushrooms and sauté for about 5 minutes, or until they are soft and have released their moisture.
3. Return the beef to the skillet with the mushrooms. Add the beef broth and bring the mixture to a simmer. Reduce the heat to low and let it simmer for about 10 minutes, allowing the flavors to meld together.
4. Stir in the sour cream and continue to cook on low heat for an additional 5 minutes, or until the sauce has thickened slightly. Be careful not to let the mixture boil after adding the sour cream to prevent it from curdling.
5. Once the sauce has thickened to your liking, remove the skillet from the heat.

Nutritional values: Calories: 600, Protein: 55g, Carbs: 8g, Fat: 38g, Fiber: 1g, Sodium: 320mg

34. BBQ Chicken Thighs with Sweet Potatoes

Preparation time: 15 minutes
Cooking time: 40 minutes
Servings: 1

Ingredients:
- 2 chicken thighs, skin on
- 1 large sweet potato, peeled and diced
- 1 tablespoon olive oil
- 1 tablespoon BBQ sauce
- Salt and pepper to taste

Instructions:
1. Preheat your oven to 400°F (200°C). Line a baking sheet with parchment paper for easy cleanup.
2. Place the diced sweet potatoes on one side of the baking sheet. Drizzle with half the olive oil and season with salt and pepper. Toss to coat evenly.
3. In a small bowl, mix the BBQ sauce with the remaining olive oil. Brush this mixture over both sides of the chicken thighs.
4. Place the chicken thighs on the other side of the baking sheet, ensuring they are not touching the sweet potatoes.
5. Bake in the preheated oven for 35-40 minutes, or until the chicken is cooked through and the sweet potatoes are tender and slightly caramelized.
6. Halfway through the cooking time, flip the sweet potatoes to ensure even roasting.
7. Once cooked, remove from the oven and let it rest for a few minutes before serving.

Nutritional values: Calories: 620, Protein: 35g, Carbs: 45g, Fat: 32g, Fiber: 6g, Sodium: 320mg

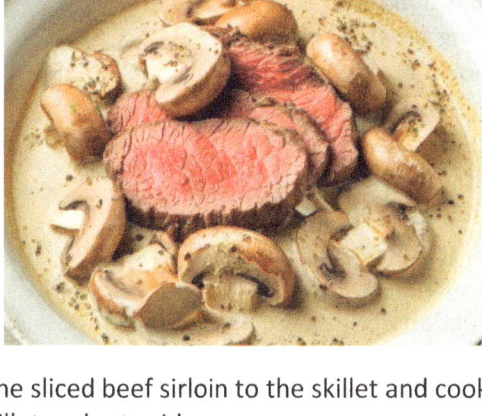

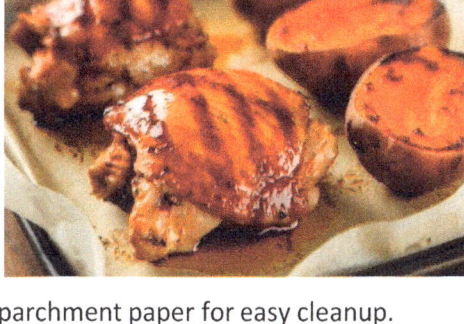

35. Lemon Herb Roasted Chicken with Asparagus

Preparation time: 15 minutes
Cooking time: 25 minutes
Servings: 1
Ingredients:
- 1 chicken breast (about 6 oz)
- 1 tablespoon olive oil
- 1 tablespoon fresh lemon juice
- 1 teaspoon dried herbs (such as rosemary and thyme)
- 1 cup asparagus, trimmed

Instructions:
1. Preheat your oven to 400°F (200°C).
2. In a small bowl, mix together the olive oil, lemon juice, and dried herbs.
3. Place the chicken breast in a baking dish. Brush the olive oil and lemon mixture over the chicken, ensuring it is well coated.
4. Arrange the asparagus around the chicken in the baking dish. Drizzle any remaining olive oil and lemon mixture over the asparagus.
5. Roast in the preheated oven for 25 minutes, or until the chicken is thoroughly cooked and no longer pink in the center, and the asparagus is tender but still crisp.
6. Check the chicken's internal temperature with a meat thermometer, which should read 165°F (74°C) when it's done.
7. Remove from oven and let it rest for a few minutes before serving to allow the juices to redistribute.

Nutritional values: Calories: 345, Protein: 35g, Carbs: 5g, Fat: 20g, Fiber: 2g, Sodium: 75mg

36. Pork Tenderloin with Apples and Onions

Preparation time: 15 minutes
Cooking time: 25 minutes
Servings: 1
Ingredients:
- 6 oz pork tenderloin
- 1 medium apple, cored and sliced
- 1/2 large onion, sliced
- 1 tablespoon olive oil
- Salt and pepper to taste

Instructions:
1. Preheat your oven to 375°F (190°C).
2. Season the pork tenderloin with salt and pepper on all sides.
3. Heat a skillet over medium-high heat and add the olive oil.
4. Once the oil is hot, add the pork tenderloin to the skillet. Sear each side for about 2-3 minutes until it develops a golden-brown crust.
5. Remove the pork from the skillet and place it in a baking dish.
6. In the same skillet, add the sliced apples and onions. Sauté for about 5 minutes, or until the onions become translucent and the apples soften slightly.
7. Arrange the sautéed apples and onions around the pork tenderloin in the baking dish.
8. Place the baking dish in the preheated oven and roast for about 20 minutes, or until the pork reaches an internal temperature of 145°F (63°C).
9. Remove the baking dish from the oven and let the pork rest for 5 minutes before slicing.
10. Serve the pork tenderloin slices with the apples and onions on the side.

Nutritional values: Calories: 600, Protein: 36g, Carbs: 18g, Fat: 44g, Fiber: 3g, Sodium: 120mg

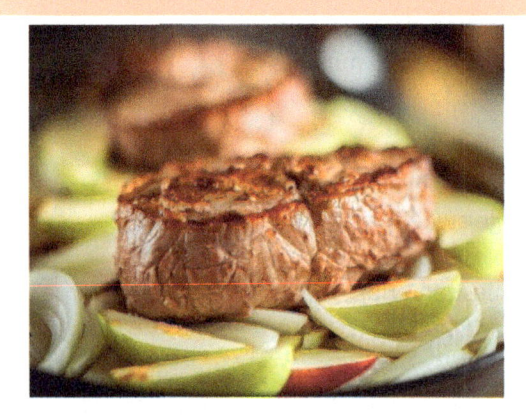

37. Shrimp Scampi with Zoodles

Preparation time: 15 minutes
Cooking time: 10 minutes
Servings: 1

Ingredients:
- 4 oz shrimp, peeled and deveined
- 2 medium zucchinis, spiralized into noodles
- 1 tablespoon olive oil
- 2 cloves garlic, minced
- 1/4 cup low-sodium chicken broth

Instructions:
1. Heat the olive oil in a large skillet over medium heat. Add the minced garlic and sauté for 1 minute until fragrant, being careful not to burn it.
2. Increase the heat to medium-high and add the shrimp to the skillet. Cook for 2-3 minutes on each side, or until the shrimp turn pink and are cooked through. Remove the shrimp from the skillet and set aside.
3. In the same skillet, add the spiralized zucchini noodles. Sauté for 2-3 minutes, just until the noodles are tender but still firm to the bite.
4. Pour the low-sodium chicken broth into the skillet with the zucchini noodles and bring to a simmer. Allow the broth to reduce slightly, about 2 minutes, which will help to flavor the noodles.
5. Return the cooked shrimp to the skillet and toss with the zucchini noodles until everything is well combined and heated through.
6. Serve immediately, ensuring a balance of shrimp and zoodles in each serving.

Nutritional values: Calories: 320, Protein: 24g, Carbs: 10g, Fat: 20g, Fiber: 3g, Sodium: 300mg

38. Teriyaki Beef Stir-Fry

Preparation time: 10 minutes
Cooking time: 10 minutes
Servings: 1

Ingredients:
- 1/2 pound beef sirloin, thinly sliced
- 1 tablespoon teriyaki sauce
- 1 cup broccoli florets
- 1 tablespoon olive oil
- 1/4 cup brown rice, cooked

Instructions:
1. Begin by heating the olive oil in a large skillet over medium-high heat. Ensure the skillet is hot before adding the beef to prevent sticking and to achieve a good sear.
2. Add the thinly sliced beef sirloin to the skillet. Cook for about 2-3 minutes, stirring occasionally, until the beef is nearly cooked through but still slightly pink in the center.
3. Pour the teriyaki sauce over the beef, stirring well to ensure each piece is evenly coated. Continue to cook for an additional 2 minutes, allowing the sauce to slightly thicken and caramelize around the beef.
4. Blanch the broccoli florets in boiling water for 2-3 minutes until tender-crisp. Drain and add them to the skillet with the beef. Toss to coat and heat through.
5. Serve the teriyaki beef and broccoli over a bed of cooked brown rice. Ensure the rice is warm before plating to keep the dish hot.

Nutritional values: Calories: 550, Protein: 40g, Carbs: 45g, Fat: 22g, Fiber: 3g, Sodium: 720mg

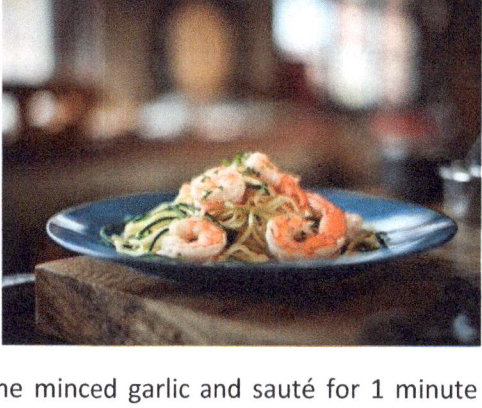

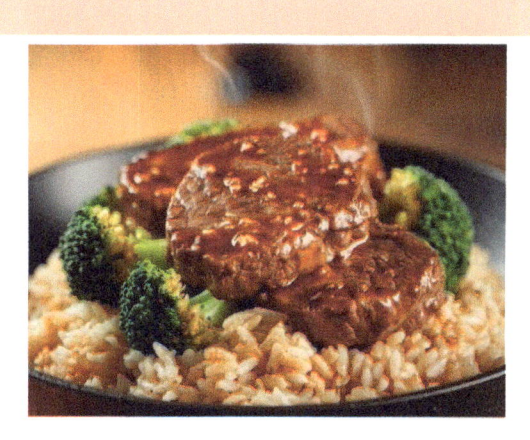

High-Calorie Snacks

39. Trail Mix Energy Bars

Preparation time: 15 minutes
Cooking time: 0 minutes
Servings: 1

Ingredients:
- 1/4 cup mixed nuts (almonds, walnuts, pecans), roughly chopped
- 1/4 cup dried cranberries
- 1/4 cup rolled oats
- 2 tablespoons honey
- 1 tablespoon peanut butter

Instructions:
1. In a medium mixing bowl, combine the mixed nuts, dried cranberries, and rolled oats. Stir these dry ingredients together until they are well mixed.
2. In a small microwave-safe bowl, combine the honey and peanut butter. Microwave for 20-30 seconds, or until the mixture is warm and can be stirred into a smooth liquid.
3. Pour the warm mixture over the dry ingredients. Stir until everything is evenly coated.
4. Line a small dish or tray with parchment paper. Transfer the mixture and press it firmly into an even layer.
5. Place the dish in the refrigerator for at least 1 hour to allow the mixture to set and harden.
6. Once set, remove the dish from the refrigerator. Lift the parchment paper to transfer the set mixture to a cutting board. Cut into bars or squares as per your preference.
7. Store the energy bars in an airtight container in the refrigerator for up to a week for quick, high-calorie snacks on the go.

Nutritional values: Calories: 420, Protein: 6g, Carbs: 50g, Fat: 24g, Fiber: 5g, Sodium: 50mg

40. Apple and Almond Butter Bites

Preparation time: 5 minutes
Cooking time: 0 minutes
Servings: 1 person

Ingredients:
- 1 medium apple, sliced
- 2 tablespoons almond butter
- 1 tablespoon granola
- 1 teaspoon honey (optional)
- A pinch of cinnamon (optional)

Instructions:
1. Start by washing the apple thoroughly. Core the apple and slice it into thin rounds for easy eating.
2. Spread almond butter on one side of each slice for a creamy, protein-rich base.
3. Sprinkle granola over the almond butter to add crunch and sweetness.
4. Drizzle a little honey over the granola if you prefer a sweeter snack (optional).
5. Finish by dusting a pinch of cinnamon over the apple slices. Cinnamon not only adds a warm, spicy note but also complements the sweetness of the apple and honey perfectly.
6. Arrange the apple slices on a plate and enjoy immediately for the best texture and crunch.

Nutritional values: Calories: 280, Protein: 4g, Carbs: 36g, Fat: 14g, Fiber: 6g, Sodium: 0mg

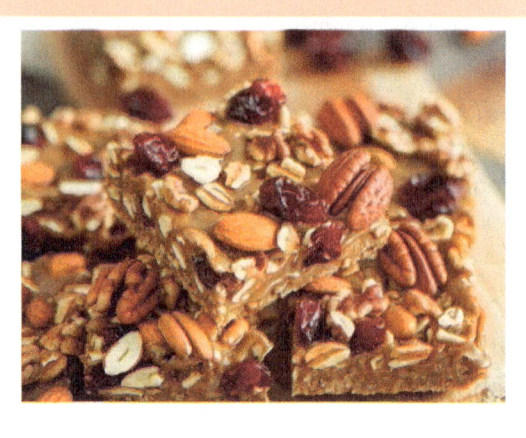

41. Coconut Cashew Clusters

Preparation time: 10 minutes
Cooking time: 0 minutes
Servings: 1

Ingredients:
- 1/4 cup unsweetened shredded coconut
- 1/4 cup cashews
- 2 tablespoons coconut oil, melted
- 1 tablespoon honey
- A pinch of sea salt

Instructions:
1. Line a small baking sheet or plate with parchment paper.
2. In a mixing bowl, combine the shredded coconut and cashews.
3. Pour the melted coconut oil and honey over the coconut and cashews. Stir until the mixture is well coated.
4. Sprinkle a pinch of sea salt into the mixture and stir again.
5. Using a spoon, scoop the mixture and form small clusters. Place each cluster on the prepared baking sheet or plate.
6. Refrigerate the coconut cashew clusters for at least 1 hour, or until they are firm.
7. Once firm, the clusters are ready to be enjoyed. Store any leftovers in an airtight container in the refrigerator.

Nutritional values: Calories: 480, Protein: 5g, Carbs: 24g, Fat: 42g, Fiber: 3g, Sodium: 60mg

42. Dark Chocolate Walnut Bites

Preparation time: 10 minutes
Cooking time: 0 minutes
Servings: 1

Ingredients:
- 1/4 cup dark chocolate chips
- 1/2 tablespoon coconut oil
- 1/4 cup walnuts, roughly chopped
- A pinch of sea salt
- 1/4 teaspoon vanilla extract

Instructions:
1. In a microwave-safe bowl, combine the dark chocolate chips and coconut oil. Microwave in 30-second intervals, stirring in between, until the chocolate is fully melted and smooth.
2. Stir in the vanilla extract into the melted chocolate mixture until well combined.
3. Fold the chopped walnuts into the chocolate mixture, ensuring they are evenly coated.
4. Line a small plate or tray with parchment paper. Using a spoon, drop dollops of the chocolate and walnut mixture onto the parchment paper, forming bite-sized clusters.
5. Sprinkle a pinch of sea salt over the top of each chocolate walnut bite.
6. Place the plate or tray in the refrigerator for at least 30 minutes, or until the chocolate has set and the bites are firm.
7. Once set, remove the dark chocolate walnut bites from the refrigerator and enjoy. Store any leftovers in an airtight container in the refrigerator.

Nutritional values: Calories: 320, Protein: 4g, Carbs: 18g, Fat: 26g, Fiber: 3g, Sodium: 50mg

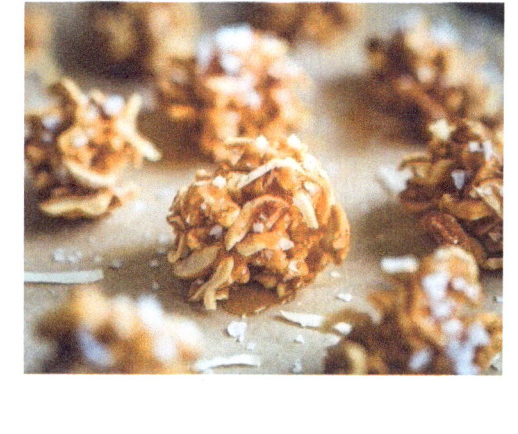

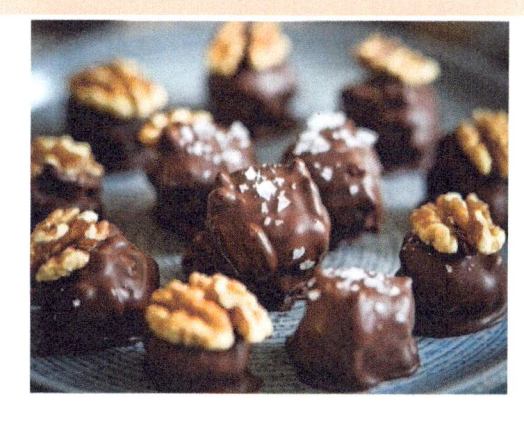

43. Greek Yogurt with Honey and Pecans

Preparation time: 5 minutes
Cooking time: 0 minutes
Servings: 1 person

Ingredients:
- 1 cup Greek yogurt, full-fat
- 2 tablespoons honey
- 1/4 cup pecans, chopped
- A pinch of cinnamon (optional for added flavor)

Instructions:
1. Place the Greek yogurt in a serving bowl.
2. Drizzle the honey evenly over the yogurt.
3. Sprinkle the chopped pecans on top of the honey.
4. For an added touch of flavor, lightly dust the top with a pinch of cinnamon.
5. Serve immediately, enjoying the mix of creamy yogurt, sweet honey, and crunchy pecans.

Nutritional values: Calories: 420, Protein: 20g, Carbs: 36g, Fat: 22g, Fiber: 3g, Sodium: 60mg

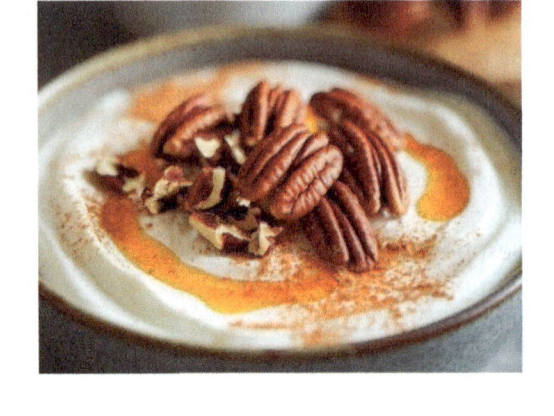

44. Peanut Butter and Jelly Protein Balls

Preparation time: 15 minutes
Cooking time: 0 minutes
Servings: 10 balls

Ingredients:
- 1 cup rolled oats
- 1/2 cup natural peanut butter
- 1/4 cup honey
- 1/4 cup dried cranberries, roughly chopped
- 2 tablespoons chia seeds

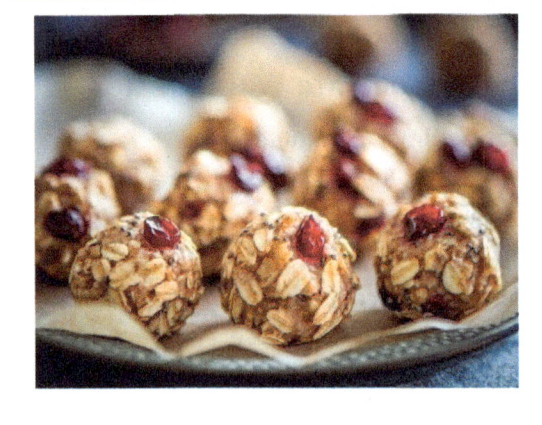

Instructions:
1. In a large mixing bowl, combine the rolled oats, peanut butter, and honey. Stir until the mixture is well combined and the oats are evenly coated with the peanut butter and honey.
2. Add the dried cranberries and chia seeds to the bowl. Mix thoroughly to ensure the cranberries and chia seeds are evenly distributed throughout the mixture.
3. Using clean hands, take a small portion of the mixture and roll it into a ball approximately 1 inch in diameter. Repeat this process until all the mixture has been used, making about 10 protein balls.
4. Place the protein balls on a plate or baking sheet lined with parchment paper to prevent sticking. If the mixture is too sticky to handle, wet your hands slightly with water before rolling each ball.
5. Once all the balls are formed, refrigerate them for at least 1 hour to set. This chilling time helps the protein balls to firm up and makes them easier to handle.
6. After chilling, the Peanut Butter and Jelly Protein Balls are ready to be enjoyed. Store any leftovers in an airtight container in the refrigerator for up to 1 week.

Nutritional values: Calories: 150, Protein: 4g, Carbs: 18g, Fat: 8g, Fiber: 3g, Sodium: 50mg

45. Cheese and Sun-Dried Tomato Crackers

Preparation time: 5 minutes
Cooking time: 0 minutes
Servings: 1 person

Ingredients:
- 10 whole grain crackers
- 1/4 cup sun-dried tomatoes, packed in oil, drained and chopped
- 1/4 cup feta cheese, crumbled
- 1 tablespoon fresh basil, chopped
- 1 teaspoon olive oil (from the sun-dried tomatoes jar for extra flavor)

Instructions:
1. Lay the whole grain crackers on a flat surface.
2. In a small bowl, mix the sun-dried tomatoes, feta cheese, and chopped basil.
3. Drizzle the teaspoon of olive oil into the mixture and stir until all ingredients are well combined.
4. Spoon the mixture evenly onto the crackers, spreading it to cover each cracker fully.
5. Enjoy immediately for a crunchy and flavorful snack.

Nutritional values: Calories: 320, Protein: 8g, Carbs: 38g, Fat: 16g, Fiber: 5g, Sodium: 520mg

46. Avocado Hummus with Pita Chips

Preparation time: 10 minutes
Cooking time: 0 minutes
Servings: 1

Ingredients:
- 1 ripe avocado
- 1/4 cup canned chickpeas, drained and rinsed
- 1 tablespoon olive oil
- 1 tablespoon lemon juice
- 1 large whole wheat pita bread

Instructions:
1. In a medium bowl, mash the ripe avocado with a fork until it reaches a smooth consistency.
2. Add the drained and rinsed chickpeas to the bowl with the mashed avocado.
3. Pour in the olive oil and lemon juice. Mix all the ingredients together until well combined and the mixture achieves a creamy, hummus-like texture. If necessary, adjust the consistency by adding a little more olive oil or lemon juice.
4. Cut the whole wheat pita bread into wedges. If desired, toast the pita wedges for 2-3 minutes in a toaster oven or on a skillet over medium heat until they are warm and slightly crispy.
5. Serve the avocado hummus with the pita wedges immediately for a fresh and satisfying snack.

Nutritional values: Calories: 450, Protein: 9g, Carbs: 49g, Fat: 26g, Fiber: 11g, Sodium: 320mg

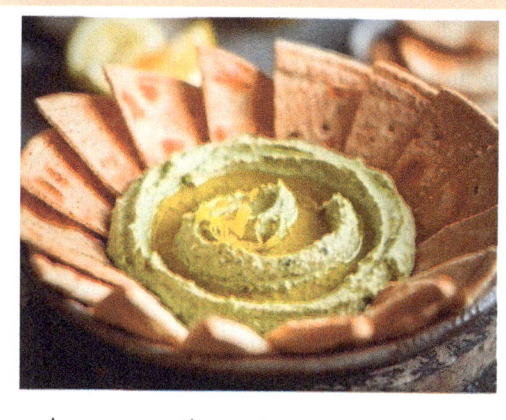

47. Banana and Nutella Roll-Ups

Preparation time: 5 minutes
Cooking time: 0 minutes
Servings: 1 person

Ingredients:
- 1 large whole wheat tortilla
- 2 tablespoons Nutella
- 1 whole banana
- 1 tablespoon chopped hazelnuts (optional for added crunch)
- 1 teaspoon honey (optional for drizzling)

Instructions:
1. Lay the whole wheat tortilla flat on a clean surface.
2. Spread the Nutella evenly over the entire surface of the tortilla.
3. Peel the banana and place it near the edge of the tortilla.
4. If using, sprinkle the chopped hazelnuts over the Nutella.
5. Carefully roll the tortilla around the banana, ensuring it is fully wrapped.
6. If desired, drizzle honey over the top of the roll-up for added sweetness.
7. Cut the roll-up in half or into smaller pieces for easier eating.

Nutritional values: Calories: 410, Protein: 6g, Carbs: 58g, Fat: 18g, Fiber: 5g, Sodium: 200mg

48. Roasted Chickpeas with Parmesan

Preparation time: 10 minutes
Cooking time: 40 minutes
Servings: 1

Ingredients:
- 1/2 cup chickpeas, drained and rinsed
- 1 tablespoon olive oil
- 1/4 teaspoon salt
- 1/4 teaspoon garlic powder
- 2 tablespoons grated Parmesan cheese

Instructions:
1. Preheat your oven to 375°F (190°C). Line a baking sheet with parchment paper for easy cleanup.
2. Pat the chickpeas dry with paper towels, removing as much moisture as possible. This step is crucial for achieving crispy chickpeas.
3. In a bowl, toss the dried chickpeas with olive oil, salt, and garlic powder until evenly coated.
4. Spread the chickpeas out in a single layer on the prepared baking sheet.
5. Bake in the preheated oven for 30-40 minutes, or until the chickpeas are golden brown and crispy. Shake the pan or stir the chickpeas halfway through baking to ensure even cooking.
6. Once the chickpeas are crispy, remove from the oven and while still hot, sprinkle the grated Parmesan cheese over them. Toss to coat.
7. Allow the chickpeas to cool slightly on the baking sheet; they will continue to crisp up as they cool.
8. Serve the roasted chickpeas with Parmesan as a high-calorie, nutritious snack.

Nutritional values: Calories: 290, Protein: 12g, Carbs: 33g, Fat: 13g, Fiber: 9g, Sodium: 480mg

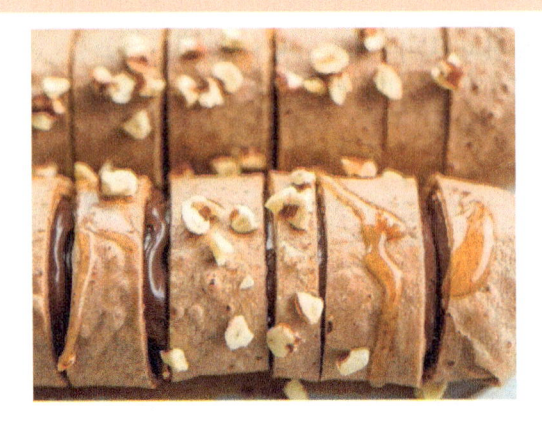

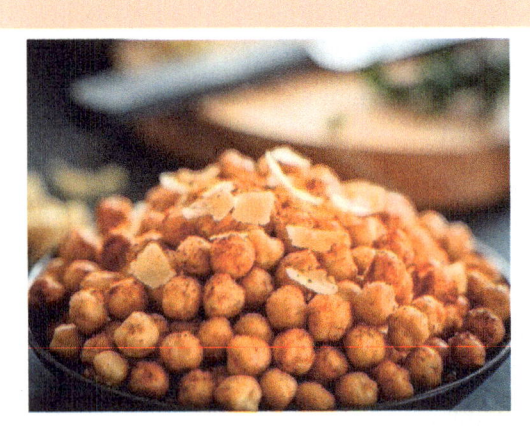

49. Almond and Cranberry Rice Cakes

Preparation time: 10 minutes
Cooking time: 0 minutes
Servings: 1 person
Ingredients:
- 2 plain rice cakes
- 2 tablespoons almond butter
- 1 tablespoon dried cranberries
- 1 teaspoon honey
- A pinch of sea salt

Instructions:
1. Spread 1 tablespoon of almond butter evenly over each rice cake.
2. Sprinkle the dried cranberries on top of the almond butter, distributing them evenly between the two rice cakes.
3. Drizzle half a teaspoon of honey over each rice cake for a touch of sweetness.
4. Finish by sprinkling a pinch of sea salt over each rice cake to enhance the flavors.
5. Serve immediately, enjoying the blend of creamy, sweet, and salty tastes.

Nutritional values: Calories: 320, Protein: 8g, Carbs: 38g, Fat: 16g, Fiber: 4g, Sodium: 200mg

50. Sweet Potato and Black Bean Nachos

Preparation time: 15 minutes
Cooking time: 25 minutes
Servings: 1

Ingredients:
- 1 medium sweet potato, thinly sliced
- 1/2 cup canned black beans, rinsed and drained
- 1/4 cup shredded cheddar cheese
- 1/4 cup salsa
- 1 tablespoon olive oil

Instructions:
1. Preheat your oven to 400°F. Line a baking sheet with parchment paper for easy cleanup.
2. Toss the sweet potato slices with olive oil in a bowl until they are evenly coated. Arrange the slices in a single layer on the prepared baking sheet, making sure they do not overlap.
3. Bake the sweet potato slices for 20 minutes, flipping them halfway through, until they are crispy and golden brown.
4. Remove the sweet potato slices from the oven and sprinkle the black beans and shredded cheddar cheese over them. Return the baking sheet to the oven and bake for an additional 5 minutes, or until the cheese is melted and bubbly.
5. Once the cheese is melted, remove the nachos from the oven. Drizzle salsa over the top before serving.

Nutritional values: Calories: 435, Protein: 15g, Carbs: 55g, Fat: 18g, Fiber: 13g, Sodium: 690mg

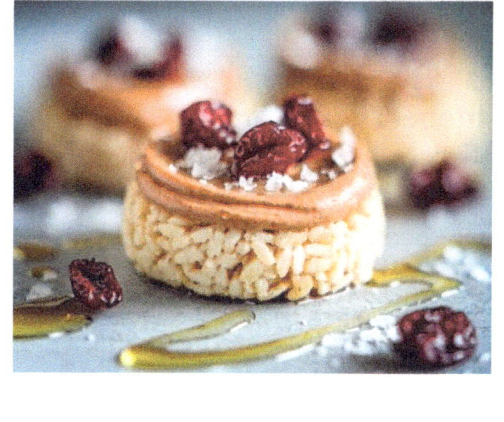

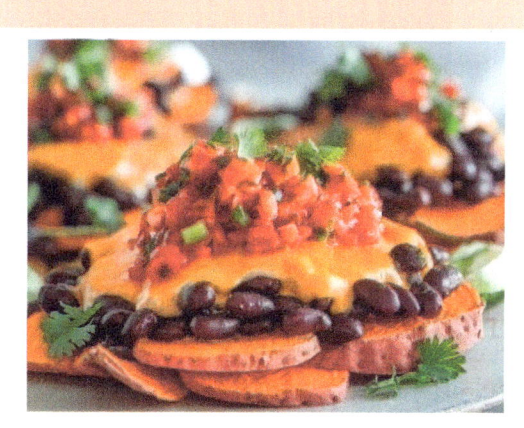

Chapter 5: Low-Calorie Day Recipes

Low-Calorie Breakfasts

51. Blueberry Almond Overnight Oats

Preparation time: 5 minutes
Cooking time: Overnight
Servings: 1 person

Ingredients:
- 1/2 cup rolled oats
- 3/4 cup unsweetened almond milk
- 1/4 cup blueberries (fresh or frozen)
- 1 tablespoon almond butter
- 1 teaspoon honey (optional for sweetness)

Instructions:
1. In a mason jar or a bowl, combine rolled oats and unsweetened almond milk. Stir until oats are fully submerged in the almond milk.
2. Add the blueberries. If using frozen ones, no need to thaw; they will defrost overnight.
3. Drop in the tablespoon of almond butter. For easier mixing, gently warm it before adding.
4. Drizzle honey over the top If desired. Adjust the amount to your taste or dietary needs.
5. Seal the jar with a lid or cover the bowl with plastic wrap. Refrigerate overnight or for at least 6 hours.
6. In the morning, give the oats a good stir to mix in the almond butter and honey thoroughly. If the mixture seems too thick, you can add a splash more almond milk to reach your desired consistency.
7. Enjoy your Blueberry Almond Overnight Oats cold straight from the fridge or let it sit at room temperature for a few minutes if you prefer it slightly warmer.

Nutritional values: Calories: 350, Protein: 9g, Carbs: 45g, Fat: 16g, Fiber: 7g, Sodium: 90mg

52. Egg White and Spinach Scramble

Preparation time: 5 minutes
Cooking time: 5 minutes
Servings: 1 person

Ingredients:
- 1 cup egg whites
- 1 cup fresh spinach, roughly chopped
- 1/4 teaspoon garlic powder
- Salt and pepper to taste
- 1 teaspoon olive oil

Instructions:
1. Heat the olive oil in a non-stick skillet over medium heat.
2. Add the chopped spinach to the skillet and sauté for 1-2 minutes, or until the spinach is wilted.
3. Season the egg whites with garlic powder, salt, and pepper. Pour the egg whites over the wilted spinach in the skillet.
4. Let the egg whites sit undisturbed for about 1 minute, then gently stir to combine with the spinach. Continue cooking for 3-4 minutes, stirring occasionally, until the egg whites are fully cooked and no longer runny.
5. Transfer the egg white and spinach scramble to a plate and serve immediately.

Nutritional values: Calories: 120, Protein: 26g, Carbs: 2g, Fat: 2.5g, Fiber: 1g, Sodium: 370mg

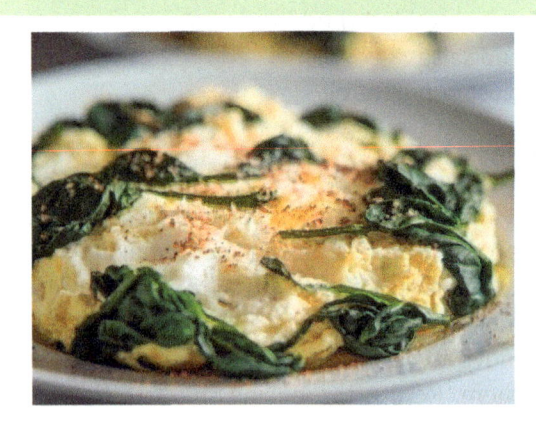

53. Cottage Cheese with Pineapple

Preparation time: 5 minutes
Cooking time: 0 minutes
Servings: 1 person

Ingredients:
- 1 cup low-fat cottage cheese
- 1/2 cup pineapple chunks, fresh or canned in juice (drained if canned)
- 1 tablespoon chia seeds
- 1 teaspoon honey (optional)
- A pinch of cinnamon (optional for added flavor)

Instructions:
1. Place the low-fat cottage cheese in a serving bowl.
2. Top the cottage cheese with pineapple chunks, distributing them evenly.
3. Sprinkle chia seeds over the pineapple and cottage cheese for added texture and nutrients.
4. If desired, drizzle honey over the top for a touch of sweetness.
5. Finish by dusting a pinch of cinnamon over the bowl for enhanced flavor.
6. Stir gently to combine all the ingredients before enjoying.

Nutritional values: Calories: 230, Protein: 28g, Carbs: 25g, Fat: 4g, Fiber: 3g, Sodium: 500mg

54. Tomato and Feta Cheese Muffins

Preparation time: 10 minutes
Cooking time: 20 minutes
Servings: 1 person

Ingredients:
- 1/4 cup whole wheat flour
- 1/4 cup low-fat milk
- 1/4 cup egg whites
- 1/4 cup diced tomatoes (drained if using canned)
- 1/4 cup crumbled feta cheese
- Non-stick cooking spray

Instructions:
1. Preheat your oven to 375°F. Lightly coat a muffin tin with non-stick cooking spray.
2. In a medium bowl, whisk together the whole wheat flour, low-fat milk, and egg whites until smooth.
3. Fold in the diced tomatoes and crumbled feta cheese until evenly distributed throughout the batter.
4. Pour the batter into the prepared muffin tin, filling each cup about three-quarters full.
5. Bake in the preheated oven for 20 minutes, or until the muffins are set and lightly golden on top.
6. Remove the muffin tin from the oven and allow the muffins to cool for 5 minutes before removing them from the tin.
7. Serve the muffins warm.

Nutritional values: Calories: 320, Protein: 18g, Carbs: 36g, Fat: 12g, Fiber: 4g, Sodium: 590mg

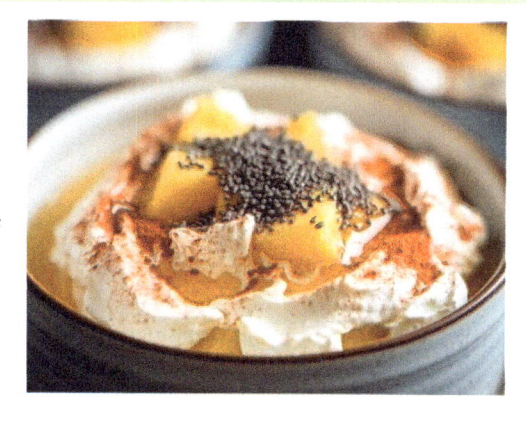

55. Cucumber and Cream Cheese Roll-Ups

Preparation time: 10 minutes
Cooking time: 0 minutes
Servings: 1 person

Ingredients:
- 1 large cucumber
- 2 tablespoons cream cheese, softened
- 1/4 teaspoon dried dill
- 1/4 teaspoon garlic powder
- 1 tablespoon finely chopped red bell pepper

Instructions:
1. Wash the cucumber thoroughly and pat it dry. Using a vegetable peeler or mandoline slicer, slice the cucumber into long, thin strips.
2. In a small bowl, mix the softened cream cheese with dried dill and garlic powder until well combined.
3. Lay the cucumber strips flat on a clean surface. Spread a thin layer of the cream cheese mixture evenly over each cucumber strip.
4. Sprinkle the finely chopped red bell pepper along the length of each cucumber strip.
5. Carefully roll up the cucumber strips tightly, starting at one end and rolling to the opposite end to create a roll-up.
6. Serve immediately or chill in the refrigerator for about 30 minutes before serving if a firmer texture is desired.

Nutritional values: Calories: 150, Protein: 2g, Carbs: 8g, Fat: 12g, Fiber: 1g, Sodium: 200mg

56. Apple Cinnamon Smoothie

Preparation time: 5 minutes
Cooking time: 0 minutes
Servings: 1 person

Ingredients:
- 1 medium apple, peeled and chopped
- 1/2 teaspoon ground cinnamon
- 1 cup unsweetened almond milk
- 1 tablespoon almond butter
- Ice cubes (optional)

Instructions:
1. Place the chopped apple, ground cinnamon, unsweetened almond milk, and almond butter into a blender.
2. Blend on high until the mixture is smooth and creamy. If the smoothie is too thick, you can add a little more almond milk to reach your desired consistency.
3. If you prefer a colder smoothie, add a few ice cubes to the blender and blend again until smooth.
4. Pour the smoothie into a glass and enjoy immediately.

Nutritional values: Calories: 215, Protein: 4g, Carbs: 29g, Fat: 11g, Fiber: 6g, Sodium: 180mg

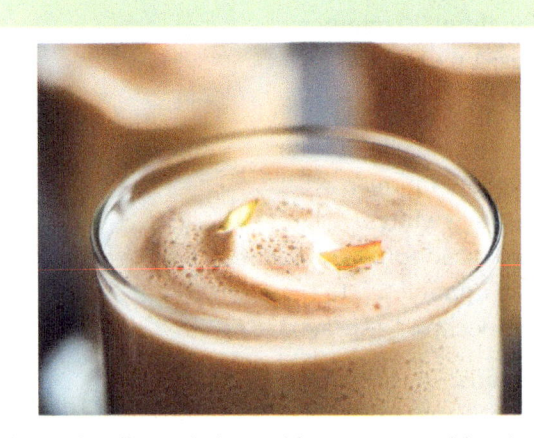

57. Avocado and Tomato Toast

Preparation time: 5 minutes
Cooking time: 2 minutes
Servings: 1 person

Ingredients:
- 2 slices of whole-grain bread
- 1/2 ripe avocado
- 1/2 medium tomato, sliced
- Salt to taste
- Ground black pepper to taste

Instructions:
1. Toast the whole-grain bread slices in a toaster or on a skillet over medium heat until they are golden brown and crispy, about 1-2 minutes on each side.
2. While the bread is toasting, peel and pit the avocado. In a small bowl, mash the avocado with a fork until it reaches a smooth consistency.
3. Spread the mashed avocado evenly over the toasted bread slices.
4. Arrange the tomato slices on top of the mashed avocado. Season with salt and ground black pepper to taste.
5. Serve immediately for a fresh and nutritious low-calorie breakfast.

Nutritional values: Calories: 250, Protein: 6g, Carbs: 30g, Fat: 12g, Fiber: 8g, Sodium: 300mg

58. Berry and Chia Seed Smoothie

Preparation time: 5 minutes
Cooking time: 0 minutes
Servings: 1 person

Ingredients:
- 1 cup unsweetened almond milk
- 1/2 cup mixed berries (fresh or frozen)
- 2 tablespoons chia seeds
- 1 tablespoon honey (optional, for sweetness)
- A pinch of ground cinnamon

Instructions:
1. In a blender, combine 1 cup of unsweetened almond milk with 1/2 cup of mixed berries. Blend on high until smooth.
2. Add 2 tablespoons of chia seeds to the blender. If you prefer a sweeter taste, add 1 tablespoon of honey. Blend on low speed just until the ingredients are mixed.
3. Pour the smoothie into a glass and sprinkle a pinch of ground cinnamon on top for added flavor.
4. Let the smoothie sit for a few minutes before drinking, allowing the chia seeds to swell and thicken the smoothie.

Nutritional values: Calories: 210, Protein: 4g, Carbs: 29g, Fat: 9g, Fiber: 10g, Sodium: 180mg

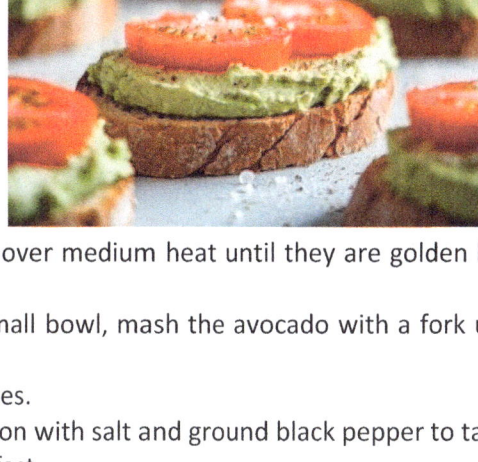

59. Egg and Avocado Breakfast Wrap

Preparation time: 5 minutes
Cooking time: 5 minutes
Servings: 1 person

Ingredients:
- 1 large egg
- 1/4 ripe avocado, mashed
- 1 whole wheat tortilla (8-inch)
- 1 tablespoon salsa
- Salt and pepper to taste

Instructions:
1. Heat a non-stick skillet over medium heat. Crack the egg into the skillet and cook to your liking, either scrambled or sunny-side up, seasoning with salt and pepper.
2. Warm the whole wheat tortilla in a separate skillet over low heat for about 30 seconds on each side or until it's pliable.
3. Spread the mashed avocado evenly over the warm tortilla.
4. Once the egg is cooked, place it on top of the mashed avocado.
5. Spoon the salsa over the egg.
6. Carefully roll the tortilla to enclose the fillings, folding in the sides as you roll.
7. Serve the wrap immediately while warm.

Nutritional values: Calories: 320, Protein: 12g, Carbs: 30g, Fat: 18g, Fiber: 6g, Sodium: 420mg

60. Zucchini and Tomato Frittata

Preparation time: 10 minutes
Cooking time: 15 minutes
Servings: 1 person

Ingredients:
- 4 large eggs
- 1/2 cup zucchini, thinly sliced
- 1/2 cup cherry tomatoes, halved
- 1 tablespoon olive oil
- Salt and pepper to taste

Instructions:
1. Preheat your oven to 350°F (175°C).
2. In a medium bowl, beat the eggs until well mixed. Season with salt and pepper.
3. Heat olive oil in an oven-safe skillet over medium heat. Add the zucchini slices and sauté for 2-3 minutes, until slightly tender.
4. Add the cherry tomatoes to the skillet and cook for an additional 2 minutes.
5. Pour the beaten eggs over the vegetables in the skillet, ensuring the eggs are evenly distributed.
6. Cook on the stovetop for 2-3 minutes until the edges of the frittata start to set.
7. Transfer the skillet to the preheated oven and bake for 8-10 minutes, or until the frittata is fully set and lightly golden on top.
8. Carefully remove the skillet from the oven (remember, the handle will be hot) and let it cool for a few minutes.
9. Slide the frittata onto a plate, slice, and serve.

Nutritional values: Calories: 400, Protein: 22g, Carbs: 6g, Fat: 32g, Fiber: 2g, Sodium: 340mg

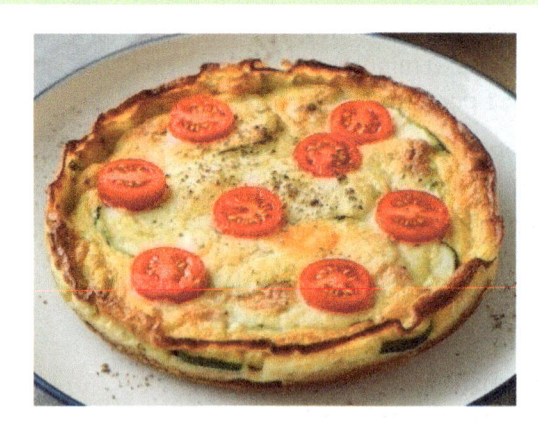

61. Raspberry and Yogurt Parfait

Preparation time: 5 minutes
Cooking time: 0 minutes
Servings: 1 person

Ingredients:
- 1 cup non-fat Greek yogurt
- 1/2 cup fresh raspberries
- 1/4 cup granola
- 1 tablespoon honey
- A pinch of cinnamon (optional)

Instructions:
1. In a serving glass or bowl, start by layering 1/2 cup of Greek yogurt at the bottom.
2. Add a layer of 1/4 cup of fresh raspberries over the yogurt.
3. Sprinkle 2 tablespoons of granola evenly over the raspberries.
4. Drizzle 1/2 tablespoon of honey over the granola.
5. Repeat the layering process with the remaining Greek yogurt, raspberries, and granola.
6. Drizzle the remaining honey on top. For a touch of warmth and spice, add a pinch of cinnamon over the final layer.
7. Serve immediately for the best combination of textures, or refrigerate for up to an hour before serving to allow the flavors to meld together more fully.

Nutritional values: Calories: 310, Protein: 25g, Carbs: 45g, Fat: 3g, Fiber: 6g, Sodium: 85mg

62. Peach and Walnut Smoothie

Preparation time: 5 minutes
Cooking time: 0 minutes
Servings: 1 person

Ingredients:
- 1 large peach, pitted and sliced
- 1/2 cup unsweetened almond milk
- 1/4 cup Greek yogurt, low-fat
- 1 tablespoon walnuts, chopped
- 1/2 teaspoon honey (optional for sweetness)

Instructions:
1. Place the sliced peach, unsweetened almond milk, and low-fat Greek yogurt into a blender.
2. Blend on high speed until the mixture is smooth and creamy.
3. Add the chopped walnuts to the blender. Pulse a few times to combine them with the smoothie without completely breaking them down, to add a bit of texture.
4. Taste the smoothie. If desired, add honey for additional sweetness, and blend again briefly to mix.
5. Pour the smoothie into a glass and serve immediately. Enjoy this refreshing, nutrient-packed breakfast that supports your metabolic confusion diet.

Nutritional values: Calories: 215, Protein: 9g, Carbs: 24g, Fat: 11g, Fiber: 3g, Sodium: 95mg

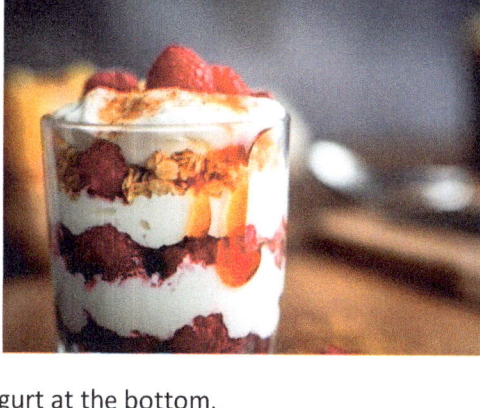

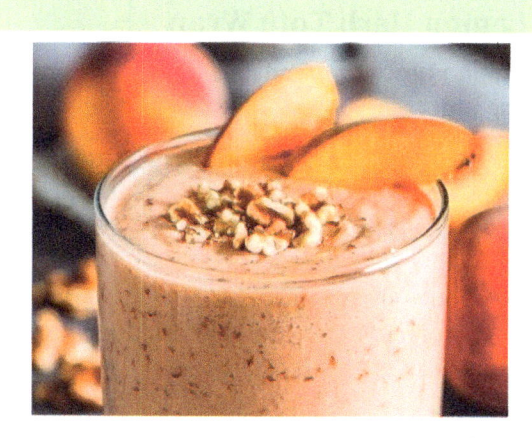

Low-Calorie Lunches

63. Grilled Vegetable and Quinoa Salad

Preparation time: 15 minutes
Cooking time: 10 minutes
Servings: 1 person

Ingredients:
- 1/2 cup quinoa
- 1 cup mixed vegetables (bell peppers, zucchini, and red onion), chopped
- 1 tablespoon olive oil
- Salt and pepper to taste
- 1 tablespoon balsamic vinegar

Instructions:
1. Rinse the quinoa under cold water until the water runs clear. In a small saucepan, bring 1 cup of water to a boil. Add the quinoa, reduce the heat to low, cover, and simmer for about 15 minutes, or until the quinoa is cooked and the water is absorbed. Fluff with a fork and set aside to cool.
2. Preheat the grill to medium-high heat. Toss the chopped vegetables with olive oil, salt, and pepper in a bowl. Transfer the vegetables to a grill basket or place them directly on the grill grates. Grill the vegetables for about 5-7 minutes, turning occasionally, until they are charred and tender.
3. In a large bowl, combine the cooked quinoa and grilled vegetables. Drizzle with balsamic vinegar and toss to combine.
4. Taste and adjust the seasoning with additional salt, pepper, or balsamic vinegar as needed.

Nutritional values: Calories: 420, Protein: 8g, Carbs: 58g, Fat: 18g, Fiber: 8g, Sodium: 200mg

64. Lemon Herb Tofu Wrap

Preparation time: 10 minutes
Cooking time: 5 minutes
Servings: 1 person

Ingredients:
- 1/2 block (7 oz) firm tofu, drained and pressed
- 1 large whole wheat tortilla
- 1 tablespoon olive oil
- 1 teaspoon dried Italian herbs (basil, oregano, thyme)
- 1/4 cup mixed greens (spinach, arugula)

Instructions:
1. Slice the tofu into thin strips. In a bowl, toss the tofu strips with olive oil and dried Italian herbs until evenly coated.
2. Heat a non-stick skillet over medium heat. Add the herbed tofu strips and cook for 2-3 minutes on each side, or until golden brown and slightly crispy. Remove from heat.
3. Warm the whole wheat tortilla in the skillet for about 30 seconds on each side, just until it's pliable and warm.
4. Lay the tortilla flat on a plate. Arrange the mixed greens in a line down the center of the tortilla.
5. Place the cooked tofu strips on top of the greens.
6. Carefully roll the tortilla around the tofu and greens, folding in the sides as you roll to enclose the filling.
7. Cut the wrap in half diagonally and serve immediately.

Nutritional values: Calories: 330, Protein: 19g, Carbs: 35g, Fat: 16g, Fiber: 6g, Sodium: 200mg

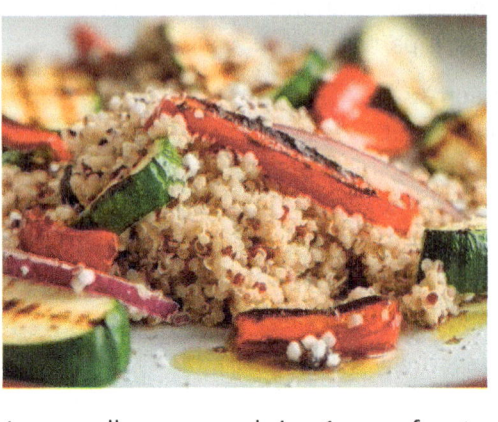

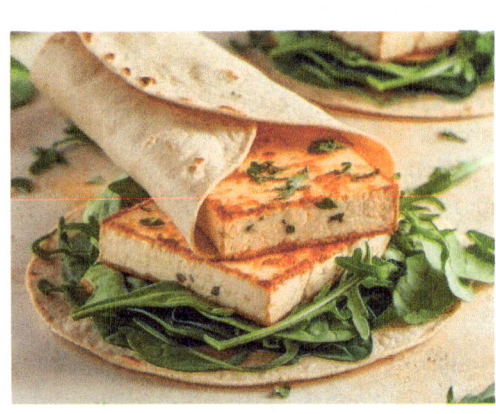

65. Cucumber and Turkey Roll-Ups

Preparation time: 10 minutes
Cooking time: 0 minutes
Servings: 1 person

Ingredients:
- 1 large cucumber
- 3 ounces of turkey breast, thinly sliced
- 1 tablespoon hummus
- 1 tablespoon feta cheese, crumbled
- 1/4 teaspoon black pepper

Instructions:
1. Begin by washing the cucumber thoroughly. Using a vegetable peeler or mandoline slicer, slice the cucumber lengthwise into thin strips.
2. Lay a slice of cucumber flat on a clean surface. Spread a thin layer of hummus over the cucumber slice.
3. Place a slice of turkey breast on top of the hummus.
4. Sprinkle a small amount of crumbled feta cheese over the turkey.
5. Season with a pinch of black pepper.
6. Carefully roll the cucumber slice into a tight roll-up. Repeat the process with the remaining cucumber slices, hummus, turkey, feta cheese, and black pepper.
7. Serve the cucumber and turkey roll-ups immediately, or chill in the refrigerator for about 30 minutes before serving if a firmer texture is desired.

Nutritional values: Calories: 150, Protein: 20g, Carbs: 8g, Fat: 4g, Fiber: 2g, Sodium: 420mg

66. Spinach and Feta Lettuce Wraps

Preparation time: 10 minutes
Cooking time: 0 minutes
Servings: 1 person

Ingredients:
- 2 large lettuce leaves (such as romaine or butter lettuce)
- 1/2 cup baby spinach, roughly chopped
- 1/4 cup feta cheese, crumbled
- 1/4 cup red bell pepper, thinly sliced
- 2 tablespoons balsamic vinaigrette

Instructions:
1. Wash the lettuce leaves gently and pat them dry with a paper towel to remove any excess moisture. These will serve as the wraps for your filling.
2. In a mixing bowl, combine the chopped baby spinach, crumbled feta cheese, and thinly sliced red bell pepper. Toss these ingredients together until they are well mixed.
3. Drizzle the balsamic vinaigrette over the spinach, feta, and bell pepper mixture. Stir the mixture again to ensure that the dressing evenly coats the ingredients.
4. Lay the lettuce leaves flat on a plate. Spoon half of the spinach, feta, and bell pepper mixture into the center of each lettuce leaf.
5. Carefully fold the sides of the lettuce leaf inwards, then roll it up from one end to the other to enclose the filling, similar to making a burrito.
6. Serve immediately, enjoying the crisp freshness of the lettuce with the tangy and savory filling.

Nutritional values: Calories: 180, Protein: 7g, Carbs: 12g, Fat: 12g, Fiber: 3g, Sodium: 420mg

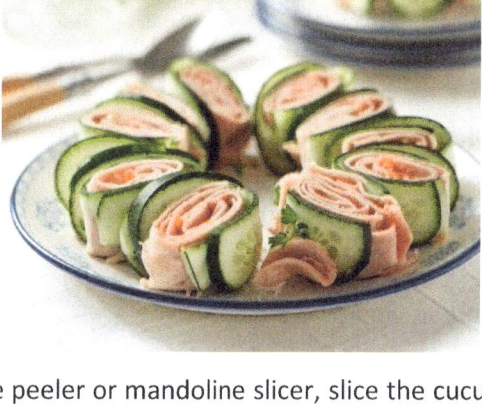

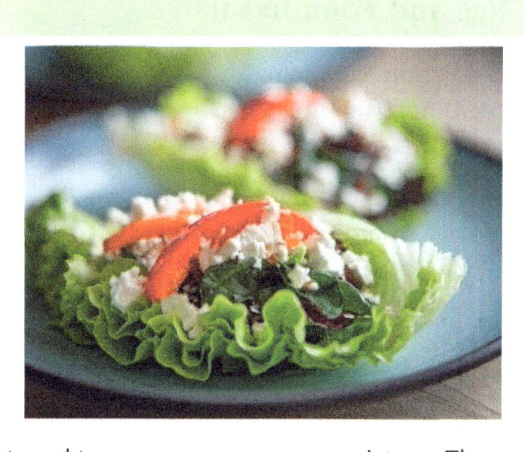

67. Tuna and Cucumber Salad

Preparation time: 10 minutes
Cooking time: 0 minutes
Servings: 1 person

Ingredients:
- 1 can (5 ounces) tuna in water, drained
- 1 large cucumber, thinly sliced
- 1 tablespoon olive oil
- 1 tablespoon lemon juice
- Salt and pepper to taste

Instructions:
1. In a medium mixing bowl, combine the drained tuna, olive oil, and lemon juice. Stir until the tuna is evenly coated with the oil and lemon juice.
2. Season the mixture with salt and pepper according to your taste preferences. Mix well to ensure the seasoning is evenly distributed.
3. Arrange the thinly sliced cucumber on a plate or in a shallow bowl to form a bed for the tuna salad.
4. Spoon the tuna mixture over the cucumber slices, spreading it evenly to cover them.
5. Optional: For an added touch of freshness, you can garnish the salad with additional lemon zest or a sprinkle of fresh herbs, such as dill or parsley, if desired.

Nutritional values: Calories: 220, Protein: 25g, Carbs: 6g, Fat: 11g, Fiber: 1g, Sodium: 390mg

68. Egg and Tomato Salad

Preparation time: 10 minutes
Cooking time: 0 minutes
Servings: 1 person

Ingredients:
- 4 large eggs, hard-boiled and peeled
- 1 medium tomato, diced
- 1 tablespoon olive oil
- Salt and pepper to taste
- Fresh basil leaves (optional for garnish)

Instructions:
1. Begin by slicing the hard-boiled eggs into quarters or roughly chopping them, depending on your preference.
2. In a mixing bowl, combine the diced tomato and sliced eggs.
3. Drizzle the olive oil over the egg and tomato mixture. Gently toss to ensure the ingredients are evenly coated.
4. Season with salt and pepper to taste. Mix lightly to distribute the seasoning without breaking the eggs too much.
5. If desired, tear a few fresh basil leaves and sprinkle them over the salad for a burst of flavor and a pop of color.
6. Serve the salad immediately, or chill in the refrigerator for about 30 minutes before serving for a refreshing and light lunch option.

Nutritional values: Calories: 320, Protein: 20g, Carbs: 4g, Fat: 25g, Fiber: 1g, Sodium: 220mg

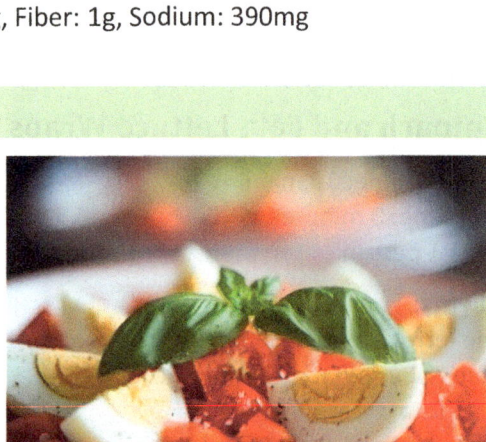

69. Zucchini and Hummus Wrap

Preparation time: 10 minutes
Cooking time: 0 minutes
Servings: 1 person

Ingredients:
- 1 large zucchini
- 1/4 cup hummus
- 1/4 cup mixed greens (spinach, arugula, or lettuce of choice)
- 1/4 cup shredded carrots
- 1 whole wheat tortilla (8-inch)

Instructions:
1. Using a vegetable peeler or mandoline slicer, slice the zucchini into long, thin strips. You will need about 4 to 6 strips to cover the tortilla.
2. Lay the whole wheat tortilla flat on a clean surface. Spread the hummus evenly over the entire surface of the tortilla.
3. Arrange the zucchini strips over the hummus, covering as much of the surface as possible.
4. Sprinkle the mixed greens and shredded carrots evenly over the zucchini.
5. Carefully roll the tortilla, starting from one edge and rolling tightly to enclose the fillings.
6. Once rolled, slice the wrap in half diagonally with a sharp knife.
7. Serve immediately, or wrap in parchment paper for a portable lunch option.

Nutritional values: Calories: 280, Protein: 9g, Carbs: 45g, Fat: 8g, Fiber: 7g, Sodium: 320mg

70. Chicken and Avocado Lettuce Wrap

Preparation time: 10 minutes
Cooking time: 0 minutes
Servings: 1 person

Ingredients:
- 1 large chicken breast, cooked and shredded
- 1/2 ripe avocado, sliced
- 2 large lettuce leaves (such as romaine or butter lettuce)
- 1 tablespoon Greek yogurt, plain
- Salt and pepper to taste

Instructions:
1. Lay the lettuce leaves flat on a plate or clean working surface, choosing the most cup-shaped leaves to hold the fillings.
2. In a medium bowl, mix the shredded chicken breast with the Greek yogurt, ensuring the chicken is evenly coated. Season with salt and pepper to taste.
3. Arrange the seasoned, shredded chicken down the center of each lettuce leaf.
4. Add slices of avocado on top of the chicken.
5. Carefully roll the lettuce leaves to enclose the fillings, tucking in the sides as you roll to secure the wrap.
6. If necessary, use toothpicks to secure the wraps for easier handling.

Nutritional values: Calories: 320, Protein: 38g, Carbs: 9g, Fat: 16g, Fiber: 6g, Sodium: 200mg

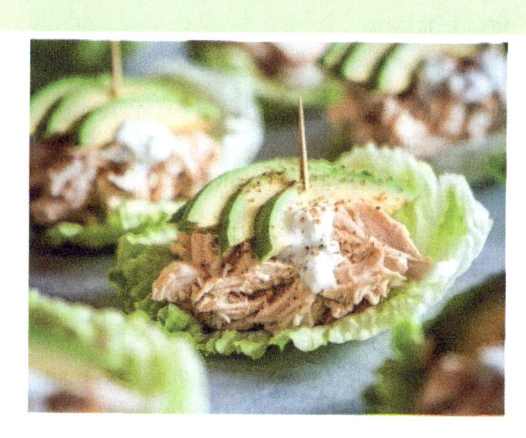

71. Cottage Cheese and Cucumber Bowl

Preparation time: 10 minutes
Cooking time: 0 minutes
Servings: 1 person

Ingredients:
- 1 cup low-fat cottage cheese
- 1 large cucumber, diced
- 1 tablespoon fresh dill, chopped
- Salt and pepper to taste
- 1/4 teaspoon garlic powder

Instructions:
1. In a serving bowl, combine 1 cup of low-fat cottage cheese with the diced cucumber.
2. Add the chopped fresh dill to the bowl. Mix well to ensure the dill is evenly distributed throughout the cottage cheese and cucumber.
3. Season the mixture with salt, pepper, and garlic powder. Stir again to incorporate the seasonings thoroughly.
4. Taste the mixture and adjust the seasoning if necessary, according to your preference.
5. Serve the Cottage Cheese and Cucumber Bowl immediately, or chill in the refrigerator for about 30 minutes before serving if a colder dish is desired.

Nutritional values: Calories: 200, Protein: 28g, Carbs: 10g, Fat: 2g, Fiber: 1g, Sodium: 500mg

72. Broccoli and Cheese Stuffed Peppers

Preparation time: 15 minutes
Cooking time: 25 minutes
Servings: 1 person

Ingredients:
- 2 large bell peppers, halved and seeds removed
- 1 cup broccoli florets, finely chopped
- 1/2 cup low-fat shredded cheddar cheese
- 1/4 cup quinoa, cooked
- 1/4 cup water

Instructions:
1. Preheat the oven to 375°F.
2. Place the bell pepper halves in a baking dish, cut-side up.
3. In a mixing bowl, combine the finely chopped broccoli florets, shredded cheddar cheese, and cooked quinoa. Mix well to ensure the ingredients are evenly distributed.
4. Spoon the broccoli, cheese, and quinoa mixture into each bell pepper half, pressing down lightly to pack the mixture.
5. Pour 1/4 cup of water into the bottom of the baking dish around the stuffed peppers. This will help to steam the peppers while they bake, keeping them moist.
6. Cover the baking dish with aluminum foil and bake in the preheated oven for 20 minutes.
7. Remove the foil and continue baking for an additional 5 minutes, or until the cheese is melted and bubbly, and the peppers are tender.
8. Carefully remove the baking dish from the oven and allow the stuffed peppers to cool for a few minutes before serving.

Nutritional values: Calories: 310, Protein: 18g, Carbs: 34g, Fat: 12g, Fiber: 6g, Sodium: 320mg

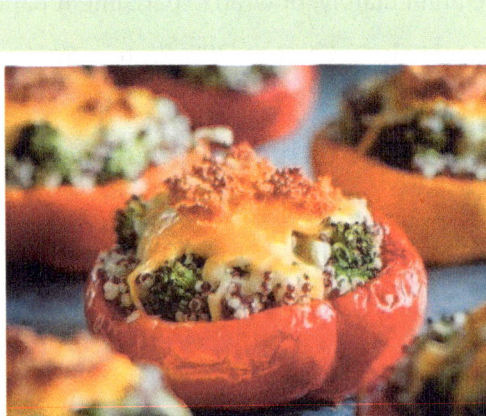

73. Tomato and Basil Salad

Preparation time: 10 minutes
Cooking time: 0 minutes
Servings: 1 person

Ingredients:
- 2 large ripe tomatoes, sliced
- 1/4 cup fresh basil leaves, torn
- 1 tablespoon extra virgin olive oil
- Salt to taste
- Ground black pepper to taste

Instructions:
1. Arrange the sliced tomatoes on a plate in a single layer.
2. Sprinkle the torn basil leaves evenly over the tomatoes.
3. Drizzle the extra virgin olive oil across the tomatoes and basil.
4. Season with salt and ground black pepper to taste.
5. Serve immediately, allowing the flavors to meld together for a few minutes if time permits.

Nutritional values: Calories: 150, Protein: 2g, Carbs: 6g, Fat: 14g, Fiber: 2g, Sodium: 10mg

74. Carrot and Hummus Roll-Ups

Preparation time: 10 minutes
Cooking time: 0 minutes
Servings: 1 person

Ingredients:
- 1 large carrot, peeled and thinly sliced lengthwise
- 1/4 cup hummus
- 1 tablespoon fresh parsley, chopped
- Salt and pepper to taste
- 1 whole wheat tortilla (8-inch)

Instructions:
1. Use a vegetable peeler or mandoline slicer to thinly slice the carrot lengthwise into long, thin strips.
2. Lay the whole wheat tortilla flat on a clean surface. Spread the hummus evenly over the entire surface of the tortilla.
3. Arrange the carrot strips horizontally across the tortilla, leaving a small border around the edges. Sprinkle the chopped parsley over the carrots. Season with salt and pepper to taste.
4. Carefully roll the tortilla tightly from one edge to the other, ensuring the fillings are securely wrapped inside.
5. Once rolled, slice the roll-up into 1-inch sections to create bite-sized pinwheels.
6. Serve immediately or refrigerate until ready to eat. Enjoy as a refreshing and nutritious low-calorie lunch option.

Nutritional values: Calories: 180, Protein: 6g, Carbs: 27g, Fat: 7g, Fiber: 5g, Sodium: 320mg

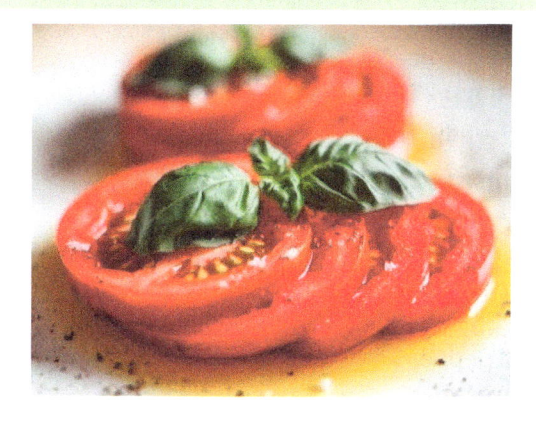

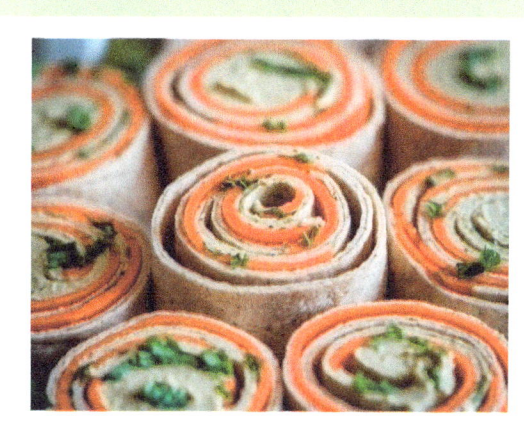

75. Eggplant and Tomato Stack

Preparation time: 10 minutes
Cooking time: 25 minutes
Servings: 1 person

Ingredients:
- 1 large eggplant, sliced into 1/2-inch rounds
- 2 medium tomatoes, sliced
- 1/4 cup low-fat ricotta cheese
- 1 tablespoon fresh basil, chopped
- Salt and pepper to taste

Instructions:
1. Preheat your oven to 375°F. Line a baking sheet with parchment paper.
2. Arrange the eggplant slices in a single layer on the baking sheet. Season both sides with salt and pepper.
3. Bake the eggplant slices for 15 minutes, flipping halfway through, until they are tender and beginning to brown.
4. Remove the eggplant from the oven. On each slice, spread a layer of ricotta cheese, then top with a tomato slice and a sprinkle of chopped basil.
5. Return the eggplant to the oven and bake for an additional 10 minutes, or until the tomatoes are just heated through.
6. Serve immediately, enjoying the layers of creamy ricotta, tender eggplant, and fresh tomato.

Nutritional values: Calories: 200, Protein: 10g, Carbs: 30g, Fat: 5g, Fiber: 11g, Sodium: 200mg

76. Cauliflower Rice Stir-Fry

Preparation time: 10 minutes
Cooking time: 15 minutes
Servings: 1 person

Ingredients:
- 2 cups cauliflower rice
- 1 cup mixed bell peppers, thinly sliced
- 1/2 cup onion, thinly sliced
- 1 tablespoon olive oil
- 1 tablespoon soy sauce (low sodium)

Instructions:
1. Heat the olive oil in a large skillet over medium heat.
2. Add the sliced onions to the skillet and sauté for 2-3 minutes until they start to become translucent.
3. Incorporate the mixed bell peppers into the skillet with the onions, continuing to sauté for another 5 minutes until the vegetables are tender yet still crisp.
4. Stir in the cauliflower rice, mixing well with the onions and bell peppers. Cook for 5-7 minutes, until the cauliflower rice is heated through and begins to brown slightly, stirring occasionally to prevent sticking.
5. Drizzle the soy sauce over the cauliflower rice mixture, stirring well to ensure even distribution of the sauce. Cook for an additional 2 minutes.
6. Remove the skillet from heat. Serve the cauliflower rice stir-fry warm.

Nutritional values: Calories: 250, Protein: 6g, Carbs: 18g, Fat: 18g, Fiber: 6g, Sodium: 510mg

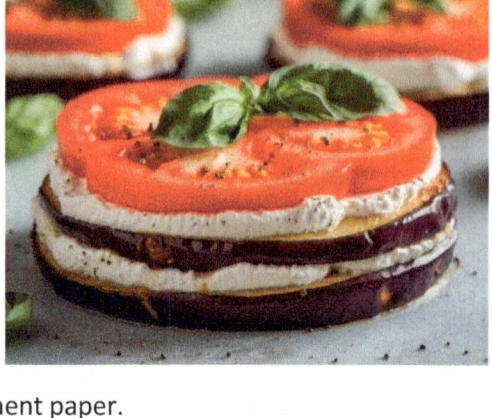

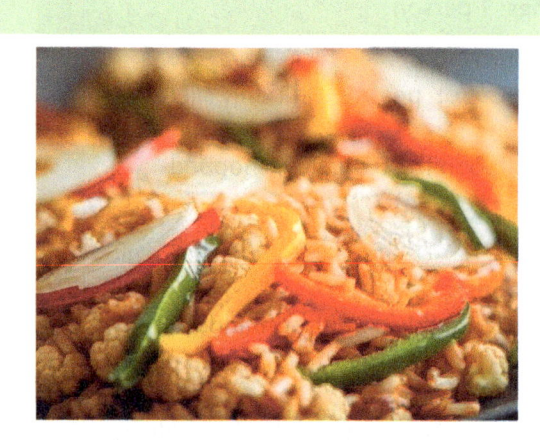

Low-Calorie Dinners

77. Grilled Lemon Herb Chicken Breast

Preparation time: 10 minutes
Cooking time: 15 minutes
Servings: 1 person

Ingredients:
- 6 oz chicken breast
- 1 tablespoon olive oil
- 1 teaspoon dried herbs (rosemary, thyme, or Italian seasoning)
- 1/2 lemon, juiced
- Salt and pepper to taste

Instructions:
1. Preheat your grill to medium-high heat.
2. In a small bowl, mix together the olive oil, lemon juice, dried herbs, salt, and pepper.
3. Brush the mixture evenly over both sides of the chicken breast.
4. Place the chicken breast on the grill and cook for about 7-8 minutes on each side, or until the internal temperature reaches 165°F and the juices run clear.
5. Once cooked, remove the chicken breast from the grill and let it rest for a few minutes before slicing. This helps to retain the juices and flavors.
6. Serve the grilled lemon herb chicken breast hot. Optional: Garnish with a slice of lemon or a sprinkle of fresh herbs for added flavor.

Nutritional values: Calories: 280, Protein: 35g, Carbs: 0g, Fat: 14g, Fiber: 0g, Sodium: 120mg

78. Baked Cod with Garlic and Lemon

Preparation time: 10 minutes
Cooking time: 15 minutes
Servings: 1 person

Ingredients:
- 6 oz cod fillet
- 1 tablespoon olive oil
- 2 cloves garlic, minced
- 1 tablespoon lemon juice
- Salt and pepper to taste

Instructions:
1. Preheat your oven to 400°F. Line a baking sheet with parchment paper for easy cleanup.
2. Place the cod fillet on the prepared baking sheet. Drizzle olive oil evenly over the top of the fillet.
3. Sprinkle the minced garlic over the cod, ensuring it's evenly distributed. Then, drizzle the lemon juice over the fillet. Season with salt and pepper to your liking.
4. Bake in the preheated oven for 15 minutes, or until the fish flakes easily with a fork and is cooked through.
5. Remove from the oven and let it rest for a couple of minutes before serving. This allows the flavors to meld together beautifully.

Nutritional values: Calories: 290, Protein: 31g, Carbs: 2g, Fat: 17g, Fiber: 0g, Sodium: 120mg

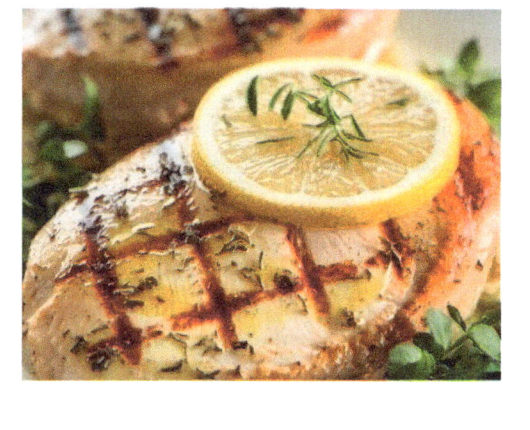

79. Spaghetti Squash with Marinara Sauce

Preparation time: 10 minutes
Cooking time: 40 minutes
Servings: 1 person

Ingredients:
- 1 medium spaghetti squash
- 1/2 cup marinara sauce, low sodium
- 1 tablespoon olive oil
- Salt and pepper to taste
- 1 tablespoon grated Parmesan cheese (optional for garnishing)

Instructions:
1. Preheat the oven to 400°F. Line a baking sheet with parchment paper for easy cleanup.
2. Cut the spaghetti squash in half lengthwise. Use a spoon to scrape out and discard the seeds.
3. Brush the inside of each spaghetti squash half with olive oil. Season with salt and pepper.
4. Place the spaghetti squash halves cut-side down on the prepared baking sheet. Bake in the preheated oven for 35-40 minutes, or until the flesh is tender and easily shreds with a fork.
5. Remove the spaghetti squash from the oven and let it cool for a few minutes until it's safe to handle. Use a fork to scrape the squash flesh into spaghetti-like strands.
6. Warm the marinara sauce in a small saucepan over medium heat until heated through.
7. Place the spaghetti squash strands on a plate. Top with the warm marinara sauce.
8. If desired, sprinkle grated Parmesan cheese over the top for added flavor.
9. Serve immediately, enjoying the comforting warmth and rich flavors of this simple, nutritious dish.

Nutritional values: Calories: 220, Protein: 4g, Carbs: 30g, Fat: 11g, Fiber: 6g, Sodium: 320mg

80. Garlic Lime Shrimp Skewers

Preparation time: 15 minutes
Cooking time: 10 minutes
Servings: 1 person

Ingredients:
- 6 oz shrimp, peeled and deveined
- 1 tablespoon olive oil
- Juice of 1 lime
- 1 clove garlic, minced
- Salt and pepper to taste

Instructions:
1. Preheat your grill to medium-high heat.
2. In a bowl, combine shrimp, olive oil, lime juice, minced garlic, and a pinch of salt and pepper. Toss to ensure the shrimp are well coated with the marinade.
3. Thread the shrimp onto skewers, leaving a small space between each shrimp to ensure even cooking.
4. Place the skewers on the grill. Cook for 2-3 minutes on each side or until the shrimp turn pink and are cooked through.
5. Remove the skewers from the grill and let them rest for a minute before serving.

Nutritional values: Calories: 240, Protein: 35g, Carbs: 3g, Fat: 10g, Fiber: 0g, Sodium: 330mg

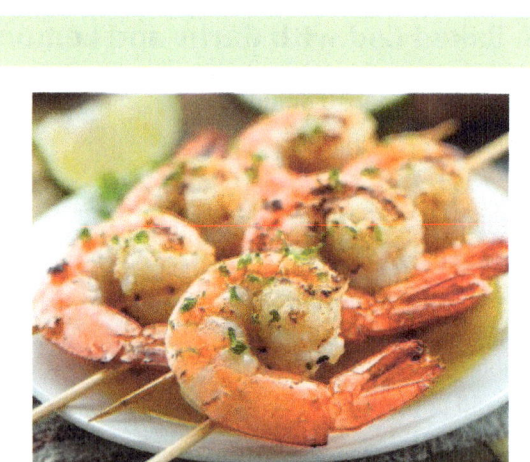

81. Turkey and Spinach Stuffed Bell Peppers

Preparation time: 15 minutes
Cooking time: 30 minutes
Servings: 1 person

Ingredients:
- 2 large bell peppers, halved and seeds removed
- 1/2 lb ground turkey
- 1 cup spinach, chopped
- 1/4 cup low-fat feta cheese, crumbled
- 1/2 cup marinara sauce

Instructions:
1. Preheat your oven to 375°F.
2. In a skillet over medium heat, cook the ground turkey until it's no longer pink, breaking it up with a spoon as it cooks, about 5-7 minutes.
3. Add the chopped spinach to the skillet with the turkey, stirring until the spinach wilts, approximately 2 minutes.
4. Remove the skillet from heat and stir in the crumbled feta cheese.
5. Place the bell pepper halves in a baking dish, cut-side up.
6. Spoon the turkey, spinach, and feta mixture evenly into each bell pepper half.
7. Pour the marinara sauce over the stuffed bell peppers.
8. Cover the baking dish with aluminum foil and bake in the preheated oven for 25 minutes.
9. Remove the foil and bake for an additional 5 minutes, or until the bell peppers are tender and the tops are slightly browned.
10. Carefully remove the baking dish from the oven and let the stuffed peppers cool for a few minutes before serving.

Nutritional values: Calories: 320, Protein: 26g, Carbs: 18g, Fat: 16g, Fiber: 5g, Sodium: 480mg

82. Zucchini Noodles with Pesto

Preparation time: 10 minutes
Cooking time: 0 minutes
Servings: 1 person

Ingredients:
- 1 large zucchini
- 2 tablespoons pesto sauce
- 1 tablespoon pine nuts
- 1 tablespoon grated Parmesan cheese
- Salt to taste

Instructions:
1. Use a spiralizer to turn the zucchini into noodles. If you don't have a spiralizer, you can use a vegetable peeler to create long, thin strips of zucchini.
2. Place the zucchini noodles in a large bowl. Add the pesto sauce to the noodles and toss gently until the noodles are evenly coated.
3. Toast the pine nuts in a dry skillet over medium heat for 2-3 minutes, or until they are golden brown and fragrant. Be sure to stir frequently to prevent burning.
4. Sprinkle the toasted pine nuts and grated Parmesan cheese over the zucchini noodles. Add salt to taste and toss everything together gently.
5. Serve immediately, enjoying the fresh and flavorful combination of zucchini and pesto.

Nutritional values: Calories: 250, Protein: 8g, Carbs: 10g, Fat: 20g, Fiber: 3g, Sodium: 580mg

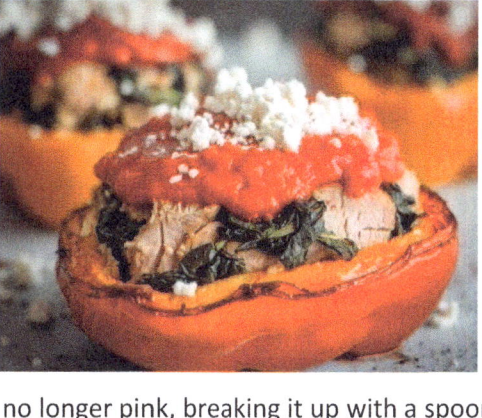

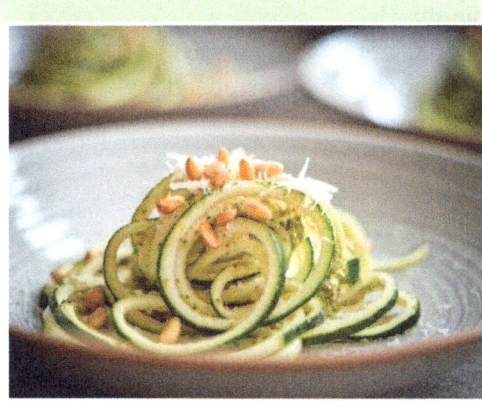

83. Grilled Portobello Mushroom Caps

Preparation time: 10 minutes
Cooking time: 8 minutes
Servings: 1 person

Ingredients:
- 2 large Portobello mushroom caps, stems removed
- 2 tablespoons olive oil
- 1/4 teaspoon garlic powder
- Salt and pepper to taste
- 1/4 cup grated Parmesan cheese

Instructions:
1. Preheat your grill to medium-high heat.
2. Brush both sides of the Portobello mushroom caps with olive oil. Season with garlic powder, salt, and pepper.
3. Place the mushroom caps on the grill, gill side down, and cook for about 4 minutes.
4. Flip the mushrooms over and sprinkle the grated Parmesan cheese evenly over the gill side.
5. Grill for an additional 4 minutes, or until the cheese is melted and the mushrooms are tender.
6. Remove the mushrooms from the grill and let them rest for 2 minutes before serving.

Nutritional values: Calories: 250, Protein: 9g, Carbs: 6g, Fat: 22g, Fiber: 2g, Sodium: 320mg

84. Lemon Dill Baked Salmon

Preparation time: 5 minutes
Cooking time: 15 minutes
Servings: 1 person

Ingredients:
- 1 salmon fillet (about 6 ounces)
- 1 tablespoon fresh dill, chopped
- 1 tablespoon olive oil
- 1/2 lemon, juiced
- Salt and pepper to taste

Instructions:
1. Preheat your oven to 375°F.
2. Place the salmon fillet on a piece of aluminum foil large enough to fold over and seal.
3. Drizzle the olive oil and lemon juice over the salmon. Sprinkle the chopped dill on top. Season with salt and pepper to taste.
4. Fold the aluminum foil around the salmon, sealing it tightly to lock in the moisture and flavors.
5. Bake in the preheated oven for 15 minutes, or until the salmon is cooked through and flakes easily with a fork.
6. Carefully open the foil packet to allow steam to escape before serving.

Nutritional values: Calories: 345, Protein: 34g, Carbs: 0g, Fat: 23g, Fiber: 0g, Sodium: 75mg

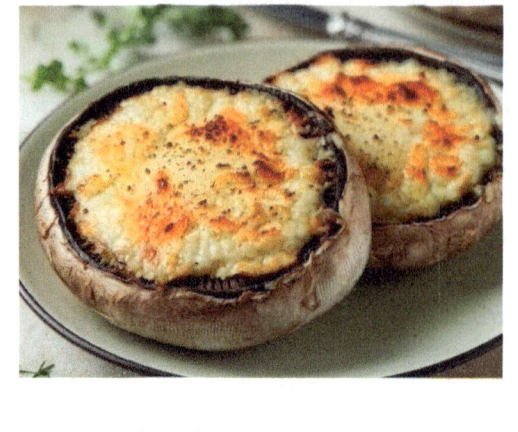

85. Chicken and Asparagus Stir-Fry

Preparation time: 10 minutes
Cooking time: 10 minutes
Servings: 1 person

Ingredients:
- 6 oz chicken breast, thinly sliced
- 1 cup asparagus, trimmed and cut into 1-inch pieces
- 1 tablespoon olive oil
- Salt and pepper to taste
- 1 tablespoon low-sodium soy sauce

Instructions:
1. Heat the olive oil in a large skillet over medium-high heat.
2. Season the chicken breast slices with salt and pepper, then add them to the skillet. Cook for about 4-5 minutes, or until the chicken is golden brown and cooked through.
3. Add the asparagus to the skillet with the chicken. Stir-fry for an additional 3-4 minutes, or until the asparagus is tender-crisp.
4. Drizzle the low-sodium soy sauce over the chicken and asparagus. Stir well to ensure the ingredients are evenly coated with the sauce.
5. Cook for another 1-2 minutes, allowing the flavors to meld together.
6. Remove from heat and serve immediately.

Nutritional values: Calories: 320, Protein: 35g, Carbs: 6g, Fat: 18g, Fiber: 3g, Sodium: 330mg

86. Cauliflower and Chickpea Curry

Preparation time: 10 minutes
Cooking time: 20 minutes
Servings: 1 person

Ingredients:
- 1 cup cauliflower florets
- 1/2 cup canned chickpeas, drained and rinsed
- 1/2 cup coconut milk
- 1 teaspoon curry powder
- Salt to taste

Instructions:
1. In a medium-sized pot, bring 2 cups of water to a boil. Add the cauliflower florets and cook for about 5-7 minutes, or until they are tender. Drain the cauliflower and set aside.
2. Using the same pot, combine the chickpeas, coconut milk, curry powder, and a pinch of salt. Stir well to ensure the chickpeas are evenly coated with the curry mixture.
3. Cook over medium heat for about 10 minutes, allowing the curry to simmer and thicken slightly.
4. Add the cooked cauliflower florets back into the pot with the chickpea curry. Stir gently to combine, ensuring the cauliflower is heated through and well-coated with the curry sauce.
5. Taste and adjust the seasoning with additional salt if needed.
6. Serve the cauliflower and chickpea curry warm.

Nutritional values: Calories: 275, Protein: 9g, Carbs: 35g, Fat: 12g, Fiber: 9g, Sodium: 300mg

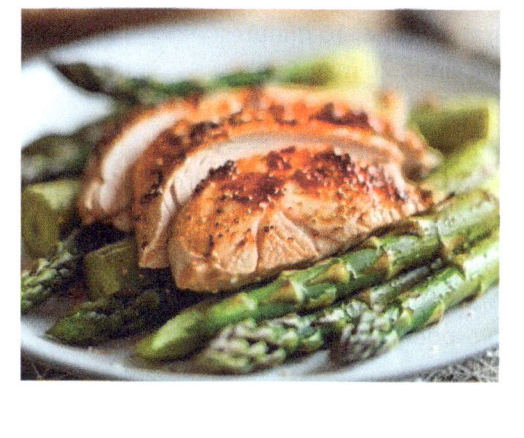

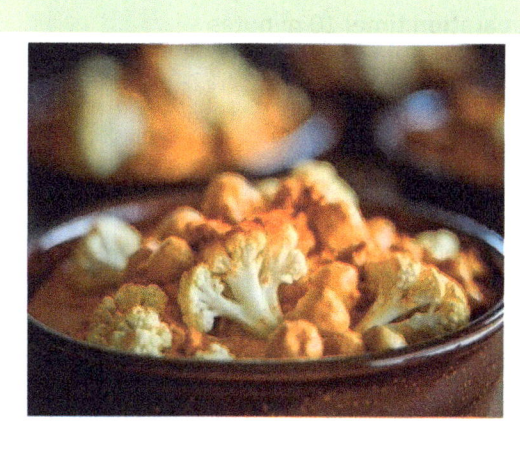

87. Balsamic Glazed Tofu with Vegetables

Preparation time: 10 minutes
Cooking time: 20 minutes
Servings: 1 person

Ingredients:
- 1/2 block (7 oz) firm tofu, pressed and cut into cubes
- 1 cup mixed bell peppers, sliced
- 1/2 cup cherry tomatoes, halved
- 2 tablespoons balsamic vinegar
- 1 tablespoon olive oil

Instructions:
1. Preheat the oven to 400°F. Line a baking sheet with parchment paper.
2. In a bowl, toss the tofu cubes with 1 tablespoon of balsamic vinegar, ensuring each piece is evenly coated. Spread the tofu cubes on half of the prepared baking sheet.
3. In the same bowl, toss the sliced bell peppers and cherry tomatoes with the remaining tablespoon of balsamic vinegar and the olive oil. Spread the vegetables on the other half of the baking sheet.
4. Place the baking sheet in the oven and roast for 20 minutes, or until the tofu is golden and the vegetables are tender and slightly caramelized.
5. Remove from the oven and let cool for a couple of minutes. Then, gently toss the tofu and vegetables together on a plate.

Nutritional values: Calories: 350, Protein: 22g, Carbs: 24g, Fat: 20g, Fiber: 6g, Sodium: 200mg

88. Cilantro Lime Grilled Chicken

Preparation time: 10 minutes
Cooking time: 15 minutes
Servings: 1 person

Ingredients:
- 6 oz chicken breast
- 1 tablespoon olive oil
- 2 tablespoons fresh cilantro, chopped
- Juice of 1 lime
- Salt and pepper to taste

Instructions:
1. Preheat your grill to medium-high heat.
2. In a small bowl, whisk together olive oil, chopped cilantro, lime juice, salt, and pepper. This will be your marinade.
3. Place the chicken breast in a shallow dish or a resealable plastic bag. Pour the marinade over the chicken, making sure it is well coated. Let it marinate for at least 5 minutes, or for better flavor, up to 30 minutes in the refrigerator.
4. Remove the chicken from the marinade, letting any excess drip off.
5. Place the chicken on the grill and cook for 7-8 minutes on each side, or until the chicken is fully cooked through and has reached an internal temperature of 165°F.
6. Once cooked, remove the chicken from the grill and let it rest for a few minutes before slicing.
7. Serve the grilled chicken garnished with additional fresh cilantro if desired.

Nutritional values: Calories: 310, Protein: 35g, Carbs: 1g, Fat: 18g, Fiber: 0g, Sodium: 70mg

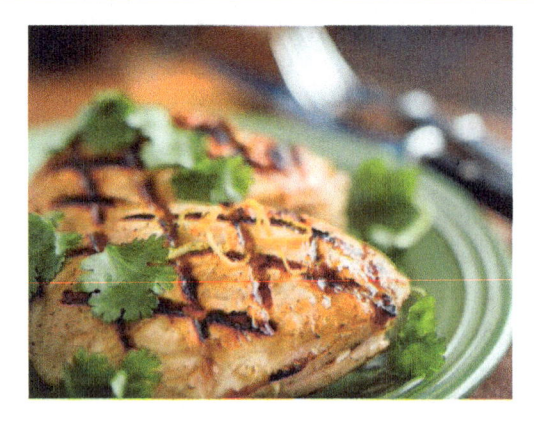

Low-Calorie Snacks

89. Cucumber and Avocado Bites

Preparation time: 10 minutes
Cooking time: 0 minutes
Servings: 1 person

Ingredients:
- 1 large cucumber
- 1 ripe avocado
- 1 tablespoon lemon juice
- Salt to taste
- 1/4 teaspoon chili flakes (optional)

Instructions:
1. Wash the cucumber and cut off both ends. Using a vegetable peeler or mandoline slicer, slice the cucumber lengthwise into thin strips.
2. In a bowl, mash the avocado until it reaches a smooth consistency. Mix in the lemon juice and salt to taste. If you like a bit of heat, add the chili flakes and combine well.
3. Lay a cucumber strip flat on a clean surface. Spoon a small amount of the avocado mixture onto one end of the cucumber strip.
4. Carefully roll the cucumber around the avocado filling, creating a small bite-sized roll. Repeat with the remaining cucumber strips and avocado mixture.
5. Arrange the cucumber and avocado bites on a plate and serve immediately.

Nutritional values: Calories: 234, Protein: 3g, Carbs: 12g, Fat: 21g, Fiber: 9g, Sodium: 10mg

90. Spicy Tuna Lettuce Cups

Preparation time: 10 minutes
Cooking time: 0 minutes
Servings: 1 person

Ingredients:
- 1 can (5 ounces) tuna in water, drained
- 1 tablespoon Sriracha sauce
- 1/4 cup diced celery
- 1/4 cup diced red bell pepper
- 4 large lettuce leaves (such as romaine or butter lettuce)

Instructions:
1. In a medium bowl, mix the drained tuna with Sriracha sauce until well combined.
2. Add the diced celery and red bell pepper to the tuna mixture. Stir until the ingredients are evenly distributed.
3. Carefully spoon the spicy tuna mixture into the center of each lettuce leaf, dividing it equally among the four leaves.
4. Gently fold the sides of the lettuce leaves over the filling, then roll them up to enclose the tuna mixture, creating a cup shape.

Nutritional values: Calories: 180, Protein: 25g, Carbs: 8g, Fat: 4g, Fiber: 2g, Sodium: 320mg

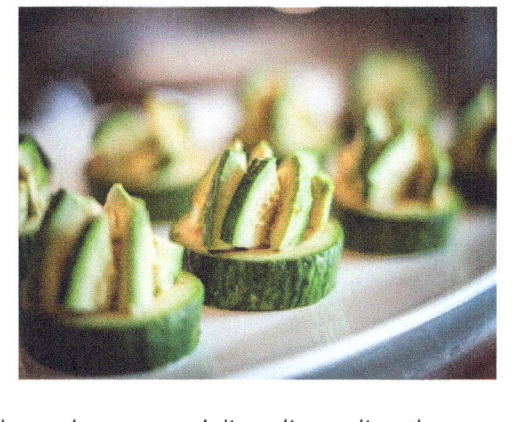

91. Roasted Red Pepper Hummus Dip

Preparation time: 5 minutes
Cooking time: 0 minutes
Servings: 1 person

Ingredients:
- 1 cup canned chickpeas, drained and rinsed
- 1/4 cup jarred roasted red peppers, drained
- 1 tablespoon tahini
- 1 clove garlic
- Juice of 1/2 lemon

Instructions:
1. In a food processor, combine the drained chickpeas, roasted red peppers, tahini, garlic, and lemon juice.
2. Blend on high until the mixture becomes smooth and creamy. If the hummus is too thick, add 1-2 tablespoons of water to reach your desired consistency.
3. Taste the hummus and adjust seasoning with salt and pepper if needed.
4. Transfer the hummus to a serving bowl. Optional: drizzle with a little olive oil and sprinkle with paprika before serving.
5. Serve with fresh vegetables or whole grain crackers for dipping.

Nutritional values: Calories: 210, Protein: 9g, Carbs: 24g, Fat: 10g, Fiber: 6g, Sodium: 320mg

92. Apple and Peanut Butter Slices

Preparation time: 5 minutes
Cooking time: 0 minutes
Servings: 1 person

Ingredients:
- 1 medium apple
- 2 tablespoons almond butter
- 1 tablespoon granola
- 1 teaspoon honey (optional)
- A pinch of cinnamon (optional)

Instructions:
1. Wash the apple thoroughly and slice it into thin rounds, removing the core with a small cookie cutter or knife.
2. Spread almond butter evenly over one side of each apple slice.
3. Sprinkle granola over the almond butter on each slice. For added sweetness, drizzle a small amount of honey over the granola.
4. Finish by dusting a pinch of cinnamon over the apple slices for a hint of spice.
5. Arrange the apple slices on a plate and enjoy as a quick, nutritious snack.

Nutritional values: Calories: 280, Protein: 4g, Carbs: 36g, Fat: 14g, Fiber: 6g, Sodium: 0mg

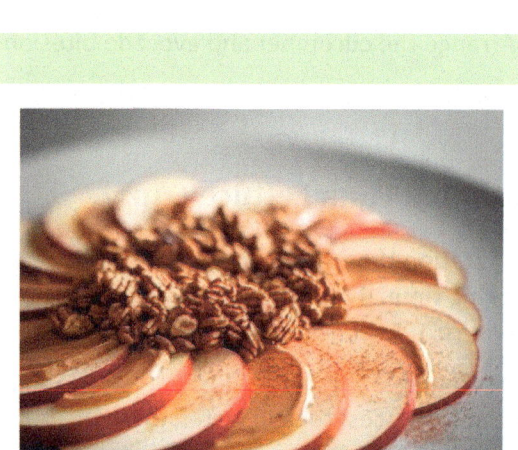

93. Celery Sticks with Cream Cheese

Preparation time: 5 minutes
Cooking time: 0 minutes
Servings: 1 person

Ingredients:
- 5 celery sticks, washed and trimmed
- 2 tablespoons cream cheese, softened
- A pinch of paprika (optional for garnish)
- A pinch of salt (optional)

Instructions:
1. Ensure the celery sticks are thoroughly washed and dried. Trim the ends to create uniform lengths.
2. Spread a generous layer of softened cream cheese over each celery stick. For easier spreading, ensure the cream cheese is at room temperature.
3. If desired, lightly sprinkle a pinch of paprika and salt over the cream cheese for added flavor.
4. Arrange the celery sticks on a plate and serve immediately as a refreshing and satisfying snack.

Nutritional values: Calories: 150, Protein: 2g, Carbs: 4g, Fat: 14g, Fiber: 1g, Sodium: 200mg

94. Cherry Tomato and Basil Skewers

Preparation time: 10 minutes
Cooking time: 0 minutes
Servings: 1 person

Ingredients:
- 1 cup cherry tomatoes, halved
- 10 fresh basil leaves
- 5 small mozzarella balls, halved
- 1 tablespoon balsamic glaze
- Salt and pepper to taste

Instructions:
1. Thread a half cherry tomato onto a skewer, followed by a basil leaf, a half mozzarella ball, another basil leaf, and finish with another half cherry tomato. Repeat this process until all ingredients are used, creating multiple skewers.
2. Arrange the skewers on a serving plate.
3. Drizzle the balsamic glaze evenly over the skewers.
4. Season with salt and pepper to taste.
5. Serve immediately as a fresh, flavorful low-calorie snack.

Nutritional values: Calories: 150, Protein: 8g, Carbs: 6g, Fat: 10g, Fiber: 1g, Sodium: 200mg

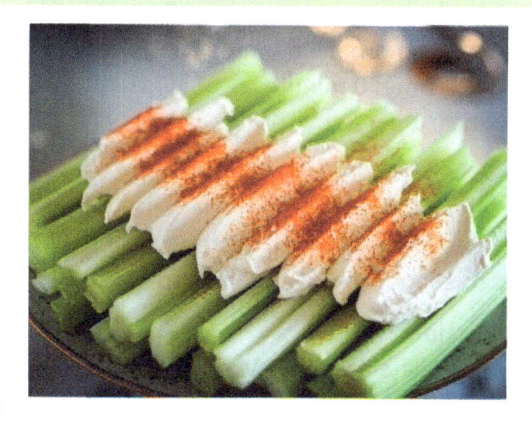

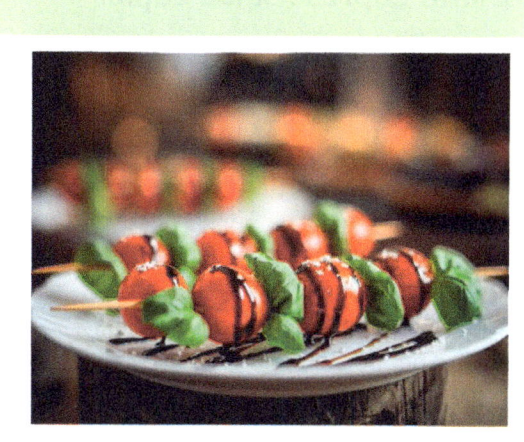

95. Almond Butter Stuffed Dates

Preparation time: 5 minutes
Cooking time: 0 minutes
Servings: 1 person

Ingredients:
- 6 Medjool dates, pitted
- 2 tablespoons almond butter
- 1 tablespoon sliced almonds (for garnish)

Instructions:
1. Carefully slice each Medjool date along one side to create an opening, making sure not to cut all the way through.
2. Spoon almond butter into the center of each date, evenly distributing the almond butter among the dates.
3. Gently press a few sliced almonds into the almond butter on each date for a crunchy garnish.
4. Arrange the stuffed dates on a plate. If desired, chill in the refrigerator for about 15 minutes before serving for a firmer texture.

Nutritional values: Calories: 320, Protein: 5g, Carbs: 54g, Fat: 12g, Fiber: 7g, Sodium: 0mg

96. Mini Caprese Salad Cups

Preparation time: 10 minutes
Cooking time: 0 minutes
Servings: 1 person

Ingredients:
- 1 large ripe tomato
- 1/4 cup fresh mozzarella cheese, diced
- 5 fresh basil leaves, torn
- 1 tablespoon balsamic glaze
- Salt and pepper to taste

Instructions:
1. Slice the tomato into 1/2-inch thick rounds and arrange on a plate.
2. Top each tomato slice with an equal portion of diced mozzarella cheese.
3. Sprinkle the torn basil leaves over the tomato and mozzarella slices.
4. Drizzle the balsamic glaze evenly across the tomato, mozzarella, and basil.
5. Season with salt and pepper to taste.
6. Serve immediately as a refreshing and nutritious snack.

Nutritional values: Calories: 150, Protein: 8g, Carbs: 8g, Fat: 10g, Fiber: 2g, Sodium: 220mg

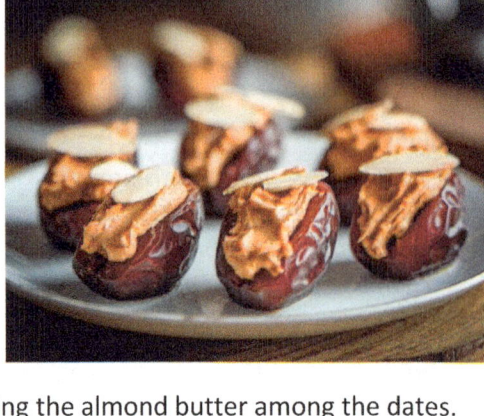

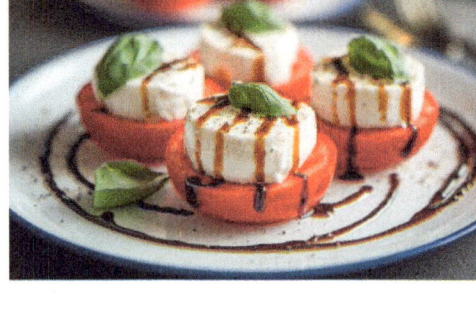

97. Kale Chips with Sea Salt

Preparation time: 10 minutes
Cooking time: 15 minutes
Servings: 1 person

Ingredients:
- 1 bunch of kale, washed and torn into bite-sized pieces
- 1 tablespoon olive oil
- 1/4 teaspoon sea salt

Instructions:
1. Preheat your oven to 300°F.
2. Place the torn kale pieces in a large bowl. Drizzle with olive oil and sprinkle with sea salt. Toss until the kale pieces are evenly coated.
3. Arrange the kale pieces in a single layer on a baking sheet lined with parchment paper, ensuring they do not overlap to promote even cooking.
4. Bake in the preheated oven for 15 minutes, or until the edges of the kale chips are slightly brown but not burnt.
5. Remove from oven and allow to cool for a few minutes on the baking sheet. The kale chips will continue to crisp up as they cool.
6. Serve immediately for the best texture.

Nutritional values: Calories: 150, Protein: 5g, Carbs: 10g, Fat: 10g, Fiber: 2g, Sodium: 150mg

98. Bell Pepper and Hummus Boats

Preparation time: 5 minutes
Cooking time: 0 minutes
Servings: 1 person

Ingredients:
- 1 large bell pepper (any color)
- 1/4 cup hummus
- 1 tablespoon diced cucumber
- 1 tablespoon diced tomato
- 1 tablespoon crumbled feta cheese

Instructions:
1. Wash the bell pepper thoroughly and pat dry. Cut the bell pepper in half from top to bottom, removing the stem, seeds, and membranes.
2. Fill each bell pepper half with hummus, spreading it evenly along the bottom.
3. Sprinkle the diced cucumber and tomato over the hummus-filled bell pepper halves.
4. Top each half with crumbled feta cheese, distributing it evenly.
5. Serve immediately as a fresh, crunchy, and nutritious snack.

Nutritional values: Calories: 180, Protein: 7g, Carbs: 20g, Fat: 9g, Fiber: 5g, Sodium: 320mg

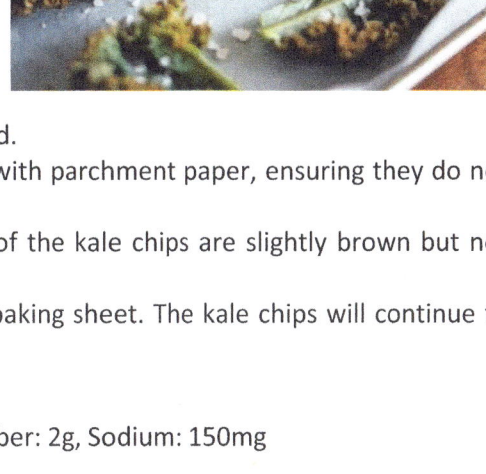

99. Greek Yogurt with Berries

Preparation time: 5 minutes
Cooking time: 0 minutes
Servings: 1 person

Ingredients:
- 1 cup non-fat Greek yogurt
- 1/2 cup mixed berries (strawberries, blueberries, raspberries)
- 1 tablespoon honey
- A pinch of cinnamon (optional)

Instructions:
1. Place the non-fat Greek yogurt in a serving bowl.
2. Top the yogurt with the mixed berries, distributing them evenly across the surface.
3. Drizzle the honey over the berries and yogurt.
4. For an added touch of flavor, sprinkle a pinch of cinnamon over the top.
5. Serve immediately, enjoying the creamy texture of the yogurt with the fresh burst of berries and the sweetness of honey.

Nutritional values: Calories: 210, Protein: 20g, Carbs: 31g, Fat: 0g, Fiber: 4g, Sodium: 70mg

100. Edamame with Sea Salt

Preparation time: 5 minutes
Cooking time: 0 minutes
Servings: 1 person

Ingredients:
- 1 cup edamame, shelled
- 1/4 teaspoon sea salt

Instructions:
1. If using frozen edamame, thaw at room temperature or in the microwave according to the package instructions.
2. Once thawed, place the edamame in a serving bowl.
3. Sprinkle the sea salt evenly over the edamame and toss gently to distribute the salt.
4. Enjoy as a nutritious and satisfying snack.

Nutritional values: Calories: 188, Protein: 17g, Carbs: 14g, Fat: 8g, Fiber: 8g, Sodium: 590mg

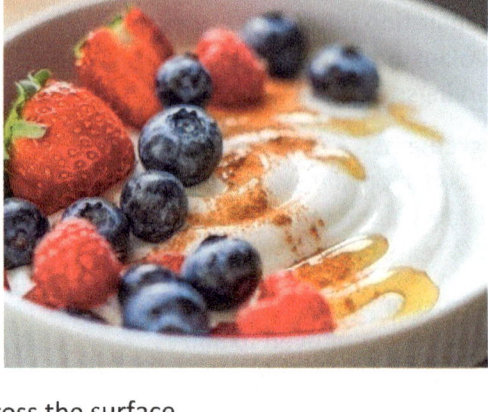

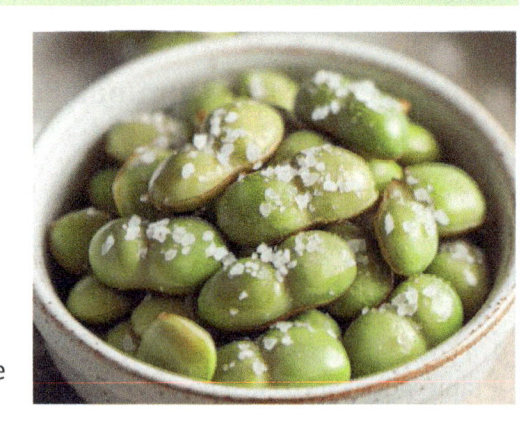

Chapter 6: The 6-Week Metabolic Confusion Plan

You've learned how metabolic confusion works—now it's time to put it into action! This **proven 6-week plan** is designed specifically for endomorph women over 50 to **ignite fat loss, balance hormones, and boost energy** without restrictive dieting. By alternating between high- and low-calorie days, your body stays in fat-burning mode while keeping your metabolism strong. This flexible plan adapts to your lifestyle, making it **easy to follow and sustain long-term**. No more guesswork—just a **clear, structured approach** to help you feel lighter, healthier, and more energized in just six weeks. Let's dive in and start transforming your health!

How to Structure a Week with Calorie Cycling

A well-balanced calorie cycling plan ensures that **low-calorie days promote fat loss**, while **high-calorie days support metabolism and muscle maintenance**. The following is an optimal schedule for women over 50 following this approach.

Sample Weekly Calorie Cycling Schedule:

- **Monday** – Low-Calorie Day
- **Tuesday** – High-Calorie Day
- **Wednesday** – Low-Calorie Day
- **Thursday** – High-Calorie Day
- **Friday** – Low-Calorie Day
- **Saturday** – High-Calorie Day
- **Sunday** – Low-Calorie Day (or Moderate Day)

This plan alternates between three **higher-calorie days** and four **lower-calorie days**, ensuring the metabolism remains active while still allowing for a controlled calorie deficit over the week. High-calorie days are best scheduled on days with higher physical activity, while low-calorie days work well for rest or lighter activity.

To help maintain long-term motivation and prevent the feeling of deprivation, you can optionally include a **moderate day** during the week. This day is designed to provide flexibility, sustain energy, and prevent excessive metabolic stress.

Key Takeaways for Weekly Calorie Cycling

- **Low-calorie days promote fat loss while high-calorie days prevent metabolic slowdown.**
- **High-calorie days replenish energy and allow for muscle maintenance.**
- **Low-calorie days should focus on lean proteins, fiber-rich vegetables, and moderate healthy fats.**
- **High-calorie days should include complex carbohydrates, healthy fats, and balanced portions.**
- **Alternating between these phases ensures sustained weight loss without the pitfalls of extreme dieting.**

By following this structured approach, endomorph women over 50 can **maximize fat loss, maintain energy, and avoid plateaus** while supporting overall metabolic health. The next step is customizing this plan to fit individual needs and preferences for long-term success.

The 4 Key Nutrients for Fat-Burning Meals

To structure meals effectively, each plate should be built around these **key nutrient categories**:

✔**Lean Proteins** – Essential for preserving muscle mass, keeping you full, and stabilizing blood sugar.
✔**Fiber-Rich Vegetables** – Helps digestion, keeps hunger at bay, and regulates insulin levels.

orts hormone balance and provides steady energy.

.tes (on high-calorie days only) – Fuels activity levels and prevents metabolic slowdown.

of these elements is what **triggers fat burning, prevents overeating, and keeps metabolism** .y.

cure for Low-Calorie Days (Fat-Burning Phase)

Low-Ca. days are designed to **create a calorie deficit while maintaining muscle and preventing energy crashes**. However, the goal is **not to starve yourself**, but rather to focus on **nutrient-dense meals** that keep you satisfied while promoting fat loss.

Guidelines for Low-Calorie Day Meals:

✔ **Prioritize Lean Protein** – Helps maintain muscle and curbs hunger (chicken, fish, tofu, egg whites).
✔ **Load Up on Non-Starchy Vegetables** – Adds volume and fiber without excess calories.
✔ **Incorporate Healthy Fats in Small Amounts** – Helps prevent cravings while keeping calories controlled.
✔ **Limit Carbs to Fiber-Rich Sources** – Stick to small amounts of quinoa, legumes, or leafy greens.

Example of a Well-Structured Low-Calorie Day:

- **Breakfast:** Greek Yogurt with Blueberries and Chia Seeds
    - o **Why?** High protein, high fiber, and low in calories to start the day right.
- **Lunch:** Grilled Shrimp Skewers with Zucchini
    - o **Why?** Protein-packed shrimp with fiber-rich zucchini for fullness.
- **Snack:** Sliced Bell Peppers with Tzatziki Sauce
    - o **Why?** A light snack that provides hydration, crunch, and gut-friendly probiotics.
- **Dinner:** Baked Cod with Steamed Asparagus and Lemon
    - o **Why?** Lean protein with detoxifying greens for a metabolism boost.

By following this structure, your body **stays in fat-burning mode while receiving essential nutrients**.

Meal Structure for High-Calorie Days (Metabolic Reset Phase)

High-calorie days **prevent metabolic slowdown and help the body recover from low-calorie days**. However, this does not mean overeating processed foods—it means **strategically increasing calories with nutrient-dense options**.

Guidelines for High-Calorie Day Meals:

✔ **Increase Protein Intake** – Helps muscle recovery and keeps metabolism active.
✔ **Add Complex Carbohydrates** – Provides sustainable energy and prevents cravings.
✔ **Include More Healthy Fats** – Supports hormone balance and satiety.
✔ **Maintain Fiber Intake** – Prevents blood sugar spikes and keeps digestion smooth.

Example of a Well-Structured High-Calorie Day:

- **Breakfast:** Whole Grain Pancakes with Maple Syrup and Almond Butter
    - o **Why?** A balanced mix of complex carbs, protein, and healthy fats for sustained energy.
- **Lunch:** Quinoa Bowl with Roasted Veggies and Hummus
    - o **Why?** High in fiber and plant-based protein to maintain fullness.
- **Snack:** Peanut Butter and Banana Smoothie
    - o **Why?** A nutrient-packed snack that supports metabolic function.
- **Dinner:** Grilled Pork Chops with Mashed Sweet Potatoes and Steamed Broccoli
    - o **Why?** A well-balanced meal that refuels energy and supports muscle maintenance.

High-calorie days should **support energy and muscle repair while preventing cravings on lower-calorie days**.

On **moderate days**, the caloric intake is balanced, with a slight focus on proteins and complex carbohydrates to boost energy and satiety.

Customizing the Plan for Your Lifestyle

Let's be honest—every woman's life looks different. Some may be juggling work, family, and hobbies, while others might have more time to dedicate to cooking and self-care. Your daily schedule, energy levels, and personal preferences should guide how you approach this plan. Customization isn't about bending the rules—it's about **making small adjustments that enhance your success**.

When you tailor the plan to **work with your lifestyle**, you'll stay more consistent, avoid burnout, and see **long-term results**.

Step 1: Evaluate Your Schedule and Energy Patterns

Understanding your daily routine and energy peaks will help you determine **when and how to eat optimally**. The **Metabolic Confusion Diet** includes both **low-calorie days and high-calorie days**, but you get to decide how those fit into your life.

- **Morning person:** If you have high energy in the morning, your larger meals (on high-calorie days) might work best at breakfast or lunch.
- **Evening person:** If you tend to feel sluggish in the morning but more energized later in the day, save your main meals for dinner.
- **Busy weekdays:** If work or family obligations dominate your weekdays, plan for **simple, grab-and-go meals** on those days. Reserve more **involved recipes** for weekends.

Pro Tip: Use the provided meal planners to schedule meals around your busiest times, ensuring you always have options ready when hunger hits.

Step 2: Choose the Right High and Low-Calorie Days

The weekly calorie cycling approach can be **adjusted to your personal needs and goals**. Here's how to customize it:

- **Athletic or physically active:** You may benefit from scheduling **high-calorie days** on days when you work out or engage in high-intensity activities.
- **Sedentary or light activity:** If you have mostly desk work or sedentary days, consider having **low-calorie days** during the workweek and **high-calorie days on weekends** when you're more active.
- **Special occasions:** Don't stress if you have a holiday, family dinner, or social event during the week. Schedule your high-calorie day around it and focus on **nutrient-dense choices**.

Pro Tip: Flexibility is key. If an unplanned event pops up, don't worry. Just adjust your high and low-calorie days to fit your week's demands. Consistency over time matters more than perfection.

Step 3: Tailor Meals to Your Tastes and Dietary Needs

Eating foods you enjoy is critical to sticking to any plan. You don't have to follow the meal plan exactly as written if certain ingredients or meals don't fit your preferences.

Here's how to personalize your meals while staying within the framework of the Metabolic Confusion Diet:

- **Allergies or sensitivities:** Swap out ingredients like dairy, gluten, or nuts for alternatives (e.g., almond milk instead of regular milk, quinoa instead of rice).
- **Vegetarian or plant-based:** Replace animal proteins with plant-based options like chickpeas, lentils, tofu, or tempeh, ensuring you meet your protein needs.
- **Flavor preferences:** Adjust spices and seasonings to your liking. If you love heat, add chili flakes to recipes. Prefer mild flavors? Use herbs like basil and parsley for a gentler touch.

- **Cultural flavors:** Incorporate your favorite cultural dishes into the plan, such as a quinoa bowl with Mediterranean flavors or a Mexican-inspired taco bowl using lean turkey.

Pro Tip: Don't be afraid to get creative. As long as you stick to the **calorie targets** for each day, you have the freedom to experiment.

Step 4: Manage Time with Meal Prep and Batch Cooking

Time constraints are one of the biggest reasons people fall off meal plans. Customizing the Metabolic Confusion Diet to fit your time limitations is crucial for long-term success.

- **Batch cook on weekends:** Dedicate 1-2 hours to preparing staples like grilled chicken, quinoa, roasted vegetables, and boiled eggs that can be used throughout the week.
- **Freeze leftovers:** Double the recipe when making dinners and freeze portions for quick meals on busy days.
- **Prep grab-and-go snacks:** Cut veggies, portion out hummus, or prepare yogurt parfaits for easy access when hunger strikes.

Pro Tip: Make use of the "5-Ingredient Recipes" in this book, which are specifically designed for quick preparation and minimal clean-up.

Step 5: Adapt for Family Meals and Social Events

One common concern for women is how to balance their diet plan with family meals or social gatherings. The good news? The Metabolic Confusion Diet can easily accommodate these situations.

- **Family-friendly meals:** Many of the recipes included in this book can be enjoyed by your entire family with minor adjustments. For example, if you're making a quinoa bowl, add extra toppings like cheese or avocado for family members who need more calories.
- **Eating out:** Choose lean proteins, veggies, and whole grains when dining at restaurants. Ask for sauces and dressings on the side to control portions and calories.
- **Potlucks and parties:** Bring a dish that fits your plan, so you have a healthy option to enjoy alongside other offerings.

Pro Tip: Don't isolate yourself. You can participate in family meals and events by **strategically planning high-calorie days** around social occasions.

Step 6: Monitor Progress and Adjust as Needed

Your body is unique, and what works for one person may not work for another. Regularly monitor your progress, paying attention to how you feel, your energy levels, and weight changes.

- **If weight loss stalls:** Consider adjusting portion sizes or reviewing your calorie intake. You may need to tweak the balance between high and low-calorie days.
- **If you feel fatigued:** Ensure you're getting enough protein, healthy fats, and hydration.
- **If you're seeing steady progress:** Stick with what's working, but remain flexible to make adjustments if your lifestyle changes.

The beauty of the **Metabolic Confusion Diet** is its flexibility. When you customize the plan to fit your unique lifestyle and preferences, you'll find it easier to stay consistent and **achieve sustainable fat loss**. This plan is not about perfection—it's about finding **what works for you** and adapting as needed. By making small, intentional adjustments, you can **turn the 6-week plan into a long-term lifestyle** that supports your health goals and keeps you feeling energized, confident, and in control.

The 6-Week Meal Plan

Week 1 Meal Plan

Day	Breakfast	Lunch	Dinner	Snack	Total Calories
Monday Low-Calorie	52. Egg White and Spinach Scramble (120)	72. Broccoli and Cheese Stuffed Peppers (310)	84. Lemon Dill Baked Salmon (345)	91. Roasted Red Pepper Hummus Dip (210)	1200
Tuesday High-Calorie	1. Avocado and Bacon Breakfast Wrap (450)	1. Grilled Chicken and Avocado Salad (600)	28. Creamy Shrimp Alfredo with Spinach (580)	42. Dark Chocolate Walnut Bites (320)	1720
Wednesday Low-Calorie	56. Apple Cinnamon Smoothie (215)	63. Grilled Vegetable and Quinoa Salad (420)	82. Zucchini Noodles with Pesto (250)	98. Bell Pepper and Hummus Boats (180)	1265
Thursday High-Calorie	2. Peanut Butter Banana Oatmeal (385)	20. Tuna and White Bean Salad (485)	27. Grilled Steak with Chimichurri Sauce (540)	45. Cheese and Sun-Dried Tomato Crackers (320)	1730
Friday Low-Calorie	55. Cucumber and Cream Cheese Roll-Ups (150)	64. Lemon Herb Tofu Wrap (330)	80. Garlic Lime Shrimp Skewers (240)	89. Cucumber and Avocado Bites (234)	1254
Saturday High-Calorie	7. Sausage and Egg Breakfast Bowl (580)	14. Quinoa and Black Bean Burrito Bowl (340)	29. Honey Garlic Pork Chops (495)	39. Trail Mix Energy Bars (420)	1835
Sunday Moderate	51. Blueberry Almond Overnight Oats (350)	21. Steak and Arugula Wrap (490)	82. Zucchini Noodles with Pesto (250)	43. Greek Yogurt with Honey and Pecans (420)	1510

Shopping List for Week 1

Proteins: Bacon, Beef steak, Cheese, Chicken, Egg, Egg whites, Pork chops, Sausage, Shrimp, Tofu, Tuna, White beans.
Vegetables: Arugula, Avocado, Bell peppers, Broccoli, Cucumber, Garlic, Lettuce, Mixed greens, Parsley, Red bell pepper, Red onion, Spinach, Tomato, Zucchini.
Fruits: Apple, Banana, Blueberries, Lemon.
Fats & Oils: Olive oil.
Herbs & Spices: Cinnamon, Dill, Garlic, Lime, Pepper, Salt.
Condiments & Sauces: Balsamic vinegar, Lemon juice, Red wine vinegar, Salsa, Soy sauce.
Other: Almonds, Crackers, Dark chocolate, Greek yogurt, Honey, Hummus, Oats, Peanut butter, Pecans, Pesto sauce, Quinoa, Sun-dried tomatoes, Trail mix, Walnuts.

Week 2 Meal Plan

Day	Breakfast	Lunch	Dinner	Snack	Total Calories
Monday Low-Calorie	61. Raspberry and Yogurt Parfait (310)	65. Cucumber and Turkey Roll-Ups (150)	77. Grilled Lemon Herb Chicken Breast (280)	97. Kale Chips with Sea Salt (150)	1190
Tuesday High-Calorie	10. Mushroom and Swiss Cheese Frittata (400)	19. Lentil and Kale Soup (310)	38. Teriyaki Beef Stir-Fry (550)	39. Trail Mix Energy Bars (420)	1680

Day	Breakfast	Lunch	Dinner	Snack	Total Calories
Wednesday Low-Calorie	58.Berry and Chia Seed Smoothie (210)	72.Broccoli and Cheese Stuffed Peppers (310)	84.Lemon Dill Baked Salmon (345)	96.Mini Caprese Salad Cups (150)	1215
Thursday High-Calorie	12.Turkey and Avocado Breakfast Sandwich (450)	18.Chicken and Quinoa Stuffed Peppers (560)	29.Honey Garlic Pork Chops (495)	45.Cheese and Sun-Dried Tomato Crackers (320)	1825
Friday Low-Calorie	53.Cottage Cheese with Pineapple (230)	66.Spinach and Feta Lettuce Wraps (180)	82.Zucchini Noodles with Pesto (250)	98.Bell Pepper and Hummus Boats (180)	1180
Saturday High-Calorie	7.Sausage and Egg Breakfast Bowl (580)	16.Beef and Broccoli Power Bowl (600)	28.Creamy Shrimp Alfredo with Spinach (580)	47.Banana and Nutella Roll-Ups (410)	1760
Sunday Moderate	51.Blueberry Almond Overnight Oats (350)	14.Quinoa and Black Bean Burrito Bowl (340)	27.Grilled Steak with Chimichurri Sauce (540)	42.Dark Chocolate Walnut Bites (320)	1550

Shopping List for Week 2

Proteins: Beef, Cheese, Chicken, Cottage cheese, Egg, Mozzarella, Pork chops, Salmon, Sausage, Shrimp, Turkey.
Vegetables: Avocado, Basil, Bell peppers, Broccoli, Cucumber, Garlic, Kale, Lettuce, Mushrooms, Onion, Parsley, Spinach, Tomato, Zucchini.
Fruits: Banana, Blueberries, Pineapple, Raspberries.
Fats & Oils: Olive oil.
Herbs & Spices: Dill, Garlic, Lemon, Pepper, Salt.
Condiments & Sauces: Pesto sauce, Red wine vinegar, Soy sauce.
Other: Almonds, Black beans, Chia seeds, Crackers, Dark chocolate, Greek yogurt, Honey, Hummus, Lentils, Nutella, Oats, Quinoa, Sun-dried tomatoes, Trail mix, Walnuts, Whole-grain bread.

Week 3 Meal Plan

Day	Breakfast	Lunch	Dinner	Snack	Total Calories
Monday Low-Calorie	57.Avocado and Tomato Toast (250)	65.Cucumber and Turkey Roll-Ups (150)	85.Chicken and Asparagus Stir-Fry (320)	99.Greek Yogurt with Berries (210)	1230
Tuesday High-Calorie	7.Sausage and Egg Breakfast Bowl (580)	20.Tuna and White Bean Salad (485)	29.Honey Garlic Pork Chops (495)	48.Roasted Chickpeas with Parmesan (290)	1850
Wednesday Low-Calorie	59.Egg and Avocado Breakfast Wrap (320)	66.Spinach and Feta Lettuce Wraps (180)	82.Zucchini Noodles with Pesto (250)	89.Cucumber and Avocado Bites (234)	1184
Thursday High-Calorie	6.Almond Butter and Honey Pancakes (485)	13.Grilled Chicken and Avocado Salad (600)	38.Teriyaki Beef Stir-Fry (550)	40.Apple and Almond Butter Bites (280)	1750
Friday Low-Calorie	53.Cottage Cheese with Pineapple (230)	63.Grilled Vegetable and Quinoa Salad (420)	79.Spaghetti Squash with Marinara Sauce (220)	100.Edamame with Sea Salt (188)	1058
Saturday High-Calorie	2.Peanut Butter Banana Oatmeal (385)	18.Chicken and Quinoa Stuffed Peppers (560)	28.Creamy Shrimp Alfredo with Spinach (580)	45.Cheese and Sun-Dried Tomato Crackers (320)	1735

| Sunday Moderate | 51.Blueberry Almond Overnight Oats (350) | 15.Shrimp and Spinach Stir-Fry (295) | 27.Grilled Steak with Chimichurri Sauce (540) | 42.Dark Chocolate Walnut Bites (320) | 1505 |

Shopping List for Week 3

Proteins: Beef, Cheese, Chicken, Cottage cheese, Egg, Pork chops, Sausage, Shrimp, Tuna, Turkey, White beans.
Vegetables: Asparagus, Avocado, Bell peppers, Broccoli, Cucumber, Garlic, Lettuce, Mixed greens, Parsley, Red onion, Spinach, Spaghetti squash, Tomato, Zucchini.
Fruits: Apple, Banana, Berries, Blueberries, Pineapple.
Fats & Oils: Olive oil.
Herbs & Spices: Salt.
Condiments & Sauces: Pesto sauce, Red wine vinegar, Soy sauce.
Other: Almond butter, Almonds, Chickpeas, Crackers, Dark chocolate, Edamame, Flour, Greek yogurt, Honey, Marinara sauce, Oats, Parmesan cheese, Peanut butter, Quinoa, Sun-dried tomatoes, Walnuts, Whole-grain bread, Whole-grain tortilla.

Week 4 Meal Plan

Day	Breakfast	Lunch	Dinner	Snack	Total Calories
Monday Low-Calorie	62.Peach and Walnut Smoothie (215)	72.Broccoli and Cheese Stuffed Peppers (310)	80.Garlic Lime Shrimp Skewers (240)	91.Roasted Red Pepper Hummus Dip (210)	1175
Tuesday High-Calorie	10.Mushroom and Swiss Cheese Frittata (400)	19.Lentil and Kale Soup (310)	30.Chicken Alfredo with Broccoli (785)	44.Peanut Butter and Jelly Protein Balls (150)	1645
Wednesday Low-Calorie	61.Raspberry and Yogurt Parfait (310)	64.Lemon Herb Tofu Wrap (330)	82.Zucchini Noodles with Pesto (250)	100.Edamame with Sea Salt (188)	1078
Thursday High-Calorie	9.Greek Yogurt and Granola Parfait (450)	21.Steak and Arugula Wrap (490)	27.Grilled Steak with Chimichurri Sauce (540)	42.Dark Chocolate Walnut Bites (320)	1800
Friday Low-Calorie	55.Cucumber and Cream Cheese Roll-Ups (150)	68.Egg and Tomato Salad (320)	79.Spaghetti Squash with Marinara Sauce (220)	97.Kale Chips with Sea Salt (150)	1140
Saturday High-Calorie	7.Sausage and Egg Breakfast Bowl (580)	13.Grilled Chicken and Avocado Salad (600)	32.Maple Glazed Salmon with Quinoa (560)	45.Cheese and Sun-Dried Tomato Crackers (320)	1760
Sunday Moderate	1.Avocado and Bacon Breakfast Wrap (450)	18.Chicken and Quinoa Stuffed Peppers (560)	38.Teriyaki Beef Stir-Fry (550)	49.Almond and Cranberry Rice Cakes (320)	1540

Shopping List for Week 4

Proteins: Bacon, Beef, Cheese, Chicken, Egg, Salmon, Sausage, Shrimp, Tofu.
Vegetables: Arugula, Avocado, Bell peppers, Broccoli, Cucumber, Kale, Lettuce, Mushrooms, Parsley, Quinoa, Red bell pepper, Spaghetti squash, Tomato, Zucchini.
Fruits: Cranberries, Peach, Raspberries.
Fats & Oils: Olive oil.
Herbs & Spices: Garlic, Lime, Pepper, Salt.
Condiments & Sauces: Lemon juice, Red wine vinegar, Soy sauce.

Other: Almonds, Crackers, Dark chocolate, Edamame, Granola, Greek yogurt, Honey, Hummus, Lentils, Maple syrup, Marinara sauce, Peanut butter, Rice cakes, Sun-dried tomatoes, Walnuts.

Week 5 Meal Plan

Day	Breakfast	Lunch	Dinner	Snack	Total Calories
Monday Low-Calorie	55.Cucumber and Cream Cheese Roll-Ups (150)	69.Zucchini and Hummus Wrap (280)	80.Garlic Lime Shrimp Skewers (240)	100.Edamame with Sea Salt (188)	1158
Tuesday High-Calorie	2.Peanut Butter Banana Oatmeal (385)	20.Tuna and White Bean Salad (485)	38.Teriyaki Beef Stir-Fry (550)	40.Apple and Almond Butter Bites (280)	1700
Wednesday Low-Calorie	62.Peach and Walnut Smoothie (215)	66.Spinach and Feta Lettuce Wraps (180)	87.Balsamic Glazed Tofu with Vegetables (350)	91.Roasted Red Pepper Hummus Dip (210)	955
Thursday High-Calorie	10.Mushroom and Swiss Cheese Frittata (400)	14.Quinoa and Black Bean Burrito Bowl (340)	28.Creamy Shrimp Alfredo with Spinach (580)	45.Cheese and Sun-Dried Tomato Crackers (320)	1640
Friday Low-Calorie	53.Cottage Cheese with Pineapple (230)	65.Cucumber and Turkey Roll-Ups (150)	79.Spaghetti Squash with Marinara Sauce (220)	97.Kale Chips with Sea Salt (150)	750
Saturday High-Calorie	1.Avocado and Bacon Breakfast Wrap (450)	16.Beef and Broccoli Power Bowl (600)	32.Maple Glazed Salmon with Quinoa (560)	39.Trail Mix Energy Bars (420)	1760
Sunday Moderate	51.Blueberry Almond Overnight Oats (350)	18.Chicken and Quinoa Stuffed Peppers (560)	27.Grilled Steak with Chimichurri Sauce (540)	42.Dark Chocolate Walnut Bites (320)	1770

Shopping List for Week 5

Proteins: Bacon, Beef, Cheese, Chicken, Cottage cheese, Egg, Salmon, Shrimp, Tofu, Turkey, White beans.
Vegetables: Avocado, Bell peppers, Broccoli, Cucumber, Garlic, Kale, Lettuce, Mushrooms, Onion, Parsley, Quinoa, Red bell pepper, Spinach, Spaghetti squash, Tomato, Zucchini.
Fruits: Apple, Banana, Blueberries, Peach, Pineapple.
Fats & Oils: Olive oil.
Herbs & Spices: Garlic, Lime, Pepper, Salt.
Condiments & Sauces: Balsamic vinegar, Red wine vinegar, Soy sauce.
Other: Almond butter, Almonds, Black beans, Crackers, Dark chocolate, Edamame, Greek yogurt, Honey, Hummus, Maple syrup, Marinara sauce, Oats, Peanut butter, Quinoa, Sun-dried tomatoes, Trail mix, Walnuts.

Week 6 Meal Plan

Day	Breakfast	Lunch	Dinner	Snack	Total Calories
Monday Low-Calorie	61.Raspberry and Yogurt Parfait (310)	64.Lemon Herb Tofu Wrap (330)	85.Chicken and Asparagus Stir-Fry (320)	100.Edamame with Sea Salt (188)	1148
Tuesday High-Calorie	2.Peanut Butter Banana Oatmeal (385)	20.Tuna and White Bean Salad (485)	32.Maple Glazed Salmon with Quinoa (560)	45.Cheese and Sun-Dried Tomato Crackers (320)	1750
Wednesday	62.Peach and	72.Broccoli and	82.Zucchini	98.Bell Pepper and	955

	Low-Calorie	Walnut Smoothie (215)	Cheese Stuffed Peppers (310)	Noodles with Pesto (250)	Hummus Boats (180)	
Thursday High-Calorie		12.Turkey and Avocado Breakfast Sandwich (450)	16.Beef and Broccoli Power Bowl (600)	28.Creamy Shrimp Alfredo with Spinach (580)	39.Trail Mix Energy Bars (420)	1800
Friday Low-Calorie		51.Blueberry Almond Overnight Oats (350)	65.Cucumber and Turkey Roll-Ups (150)	77.Grilled Lemon Herb Chicken Breast (280)	96.Mini Caprese Salad Cups (150)	930
Saturday High-Calorie		7.Sausage and Egg Breakfast Bowl (580)	18.Chicken and Quinoa Stuffed Peppers (560)	27.Grilled Steak with Chimichurri Sauce (540)	42.Dark Chocolate Walnut Bites (320)	1740
Sunday Moderate		1.Avocado and Bacon Breakfast Wrap (450)	21.Steak and Arugula Wrap (490)	29.Honey Garlic Pork Chops (495)	40.Apple and Almond Butter Bites (280)	1615

Shopping List for Week 6

Proteins: Bacon, Beef, Cheese, Chicken, Egg, Mozzarella, Pork chops, Sausage, Salmon, Shrimp, Tofu, Turkey, White beans.
Vegetables: Arugula, Asparagus, Avocado, Basil, Bell peppers, Broccoli, Cucumber, Garlic, Lettuce, Onion, Parsley, Quinoa, Red bell pepper, Spinach, Tomato, Zucchini.
Fruits: Apple, Banana, Blueberries, Peach, Raspberries.
Fats & Oils: Olive oil.
Herbs & Spices: Garlic, Lemon, Pepper, Salt.
Condiments & Sauces: Lemon juice, Pesto sauce, Red wine vinegar.
Other: Almond butter, Almonds, Crackers, Dark chocolate, Edamame, Greek yogurt, Honey, Hummus, Maple syrup, Oats, Peanut butter, Sun-dried tomatoes, Trail mix, Walnuts, Whole-grain bread.

DOWNLOAD YOUR EXCLUSIVE BONUSES HERE:

Or at this link: http://bit.ly/3Qbu63i

Chapter 7: Tailoring Your Calorie Plan for Maximum Results

What a typical weekly plan might look like:

Day	Breakfast	Lunch	Dinner	Snack	Total Calories
Monday					1200-1400 kcal (low)
Tuesday					1800-2200 kcal (high)
Wednesday					1200-1400 kcal (low)
Thursday					1800-2200 kcal (high)
Friday					1200-1400 kcal (low)
Saturday					1800-2200 kcal (high)
Sunday					1600-1800 kcal (moderate)

The calorie ranges I have indicated (1800-2200 kcal for high-calorie days and 1200-1400 kcal for low-calorie days) are common examples, but the precise values depend on several factors, such as:

- Age
- Gender
- Body weight and body composition
- Level of physical activity
- Specific goals (weight loss, maintenance, etc.)

Therefore, these ranges are indicative and represent an average for the general population. They can be adjusted based on individual needs.

How to calculate your personal ranges

One way to establish your ranges is to calculate your **total daily energy expenditure (TDEE)**, which represents the number of calories your body needs to maintain its current weight.

How to calculate TDEE (Total Daily Energy Expenditure)

TDEE is the **total amount of calories you burn in a day**, including everything from resting metabolism (energy needed for basic body functions) to physical activity.

It is calculated by first determining your **Basal Metabolic Rate (BMR)** and then multiplying it by an **activity factor** that reflects your daily activity level.

Step 1: Calculate BMR (Basal Metabolic Rate)

The most common formulas for calculating BMR are the **Mifflin-St Jeor Equation** and the **Harris-Benedict Equation**. The Mifflin-St Jeor Equation is generally more accurate.

Mifflin-St Jeor Equation:

- For women:

    BMR = 655 + (4.35 × weight in lbs) + (4.7 × height in inches) − (4.7 × age in years)

- For men:

    BMR = 66 + (6.23 × weight in lbs) + (12.7 × height in inches) − (6.8 × age in years)

Example Calculation:

- Female, 55 years old, 154 lbs, 65 inches (5'5")

    BMR = 655 + (4.35 × 154) + (4.7 × 65) − (4.7 × 55) = 655 + 669.9 + 305.5 − 258.5 = 1372 kcal/day

Step 2: Multiply BMR by an Activity Factor

Choose an activity factor that reflects your lifestyle:

Activity Level	Activity Factor	Description
Sedentary (little/no exercise)	1.2	Office work, little physical activity
Lightly active	1.375	Light exercise/sports 1-3 days per week
Moderately active	1.55	Moderate exercise/sports 3-5 days per week
Very active	1.725	Hard exercise/sports 6-7 days per week
Extremely active	1.9	Very intense exercise, physical labor, or training twice daily

Example (lightly active female, 55 years old):

TDEE = 1372 × 1.375 = 1885 kcal/day

Online TDEE Calculators

If you don't want to calculate it manually, there are several free online calculators that use the Mifflin-St Jeor Equation and apply the correct activity factor.

Step 3: Adjust TDEE Based on Goals

- **For weight loss:** Create a deficit of 10-20% from your TDEE.
  Example: 1885 kcal/day → 1500-1700 kcal for low-calorie days.
- **For maintenance:** Stick close to your TDEE.
- **For muscle gain:** Add 10-15% more calories than TDEE.

Step 4: Determine Your High and Low-Calorie Days

Once you have your **TDEE**, follow these guidelines:

- **High-Calorie Days:** Eat **close to your TDEE** or slightly higher (+10-15% if needed).
- **Low-Calorie Days:** Eat **70-80% of your TDEE** to create a deficit.
- **Moderate Days:** Eat **85-90% of your TDEE** to provide flexibility.

Important: Minimum caloric intake on low-calorie days

It is important that on low-calorie days you never go below your minimum caloric intake unless advised by a healthcare professional to avoid issues such as:

- Fatigue and loss of muscle mass.
- Slowing down of metabolism.
- Extreme hunger, which can lead to binge eating episodes.

How to convert between metric and imperial units:

- **To convert lbs to kg:** lbs ÷ 2.205 = kg
- **To convert inches to cm:** inches × 2.54 = cm

Tips for Success:

- **Always listen to your body:** If you feel fatigued or overly hungry, adjust your intake slightly.
- **Protein intake:** Maintain adequate protein to preserve muscle mass, especially on low-calorie days.
- **Track progress:** If you're not seeing results, consider re-evaluating your TDEE or increasing physical activity.

Chapter 8: Overcoming Challenges and Thriving Beyond the 6-Week Plan

The Metabolic Confusion Diet isn't just a temporary solution—it's a gateway to lasting health and vitality. But even the most successful journeys have their share of challenges. Weight plateaus, dips in motivation, and life's unpredictability can all test your resolve. The key is to embrace these moments as part of the process, knowing that lasting change is built on persistence, adaptability, and self-compassion.

This chapter is your guide to navigating setbacks, maintaining progress, and evolving from a structured 6-week plan into a lifestyle that feels natural and empowering. Through consistency, flexibility, and sustainable habits, you'll learn how to overcome obstacles and keep thriving long after the initial phase.

Embrace Small, Consistent Progress

Instead of focusing on perfection, prioritize small wins. Progress isn't about never slipping up—it's about always getting back on track. Prep meals ahead, stay hydrated, and schedule short daily movement. When you prioritize simple, consistent actions, progress becomes sustainable.

Calorie Cycling as a Lifelong Tool

Calorie cycling doesn't end after 6 weeks. You can adapt it based on your needs, balancing higher intake during active periods or social events and lower intake during quieter days. Listen to your body, adjust as needed, and keep flexibility at the forefront of your plan.

Break Through Weight Plateaus

When progress slows, don't panic—it's normal. Consider mixing up your routine, such as switching meal timing or adding new exercises like light strength training. Adjust your high/low-calorie days if needed to reignite results.

Nourish with Whole, Nutrient-Dense Foods

A healthy, lifelong approach is built on nourishing your body with foods that keep you energized and balanced. Stick to whole foods 80% of the time, allowing room for indulgences in moderation. Try new recipes, explore flavors, and keep meals exciting to avoid boredom.

Stay Active and Prioritize Recovery

Movement is essential for maintaining metabolism and muscle mass, but balance is key. Mix cardio, strength training, and gentle exercises like yoga or stretching. Prioritize sleep and recovery days to help your body heal and recharge.

Lean on Support and Celebrate Wins

Connect with family, friends, or online communities who understand your journey. Small wins, like better sleep or increased energy, deserve recognition. Reward yourself with non-food treats, like a new outfit or a relaxing day off.

Evolve and Adapt Over Time

As your body changes, so should your approach. Stay curious about what works, adjust your habits as needed, and be kind to yourself through it all. This is a journey of self-discovery, not a race to perfection.

By embracing these sustainable practices, you'll turn short-term progress into lifelong success. You've already taken the most important step—now, keep moving forward with confidence, compassion, and the knowledge that you're creating a healthier, more vibrant future.

Conclusion

You've made it to the end of this book, and what a journey it's been! First, let me say how proud I am of you. Just by picking up this book, you made a commitment to yourself—a commitment to prioritize your health, take control of your weight, and discover a sustainable path to feeling better in your body. And I hope you've seen that this journey isn't about perfection but about progress, one step at a time.

If you're an endomorph woman over 50 like me, you know the challenges we face aren't just about the number on the scale. It's about balancing hormones that seem to work against us, boosting our energy to keep up with family and daily life, and finding relief from the frustration of diets that don't seem to fit our unique bodies. But now, you have something different—a plan tailored to your needs, rooted in science, and designed to work *with* your body rather than against it.

This 6-week metabolic confusion plan is just the beginning. Whether you've hit every goal or are still finding your rhythm, know this: your journey isn't over. True health is built on consistency, compassion for yourself, and the willingness to keep going even when the results aren't immediate. There's no rush, no deadline, and no need to compare yourself to anyone else. Your journey is yours alone, and every small victory—whether it's a better night's sleep, more energy to play with the grandkids, or simply feeling good in your clothes—is worth celebrating.

As you move forward, remember what we've learned:

You don't have to starve yourself to see results.

High-calorie days aren't setbacks—they're part of the plan.

Simple, 5-ingredient meals can be just as satisfying as complicated recipes.

And most importantly, you have the power to achieve long-lasting change.

Even when life gets hectic or you face moments of doubt, remind yourself of your progress. Reflect on how far you've come, and if you ever feel stuck, return to these pages for guidance and motivation. Remember that setbacks are normal, and they don't define you—what matters is how you bounce back.

This book was written with you in mind. I want you to know that you're not alone on this journey. Every meal, every choice, and every effort you make toward your health is an act of self-love. And you deserve that love, always.

Thank you for letting me be a part of your transformation. My hope is that this book has not only helped you develop healthier eating habits but has also reminded you of your strength and resilience. You've got this!

Here's to a future of balanced hormones, steady energy, and feeling truly at home in your body. Take what you've learned and make it your own. Your best, healthiest life is waiting.

With love and encouragement,

Cynthia Digges

DOWNLOAD YOUR EXCLUSIVE BONUSES ON PAGE 69

Made in the USA
Las Vegas, NV
20 March 2025